resetting normal

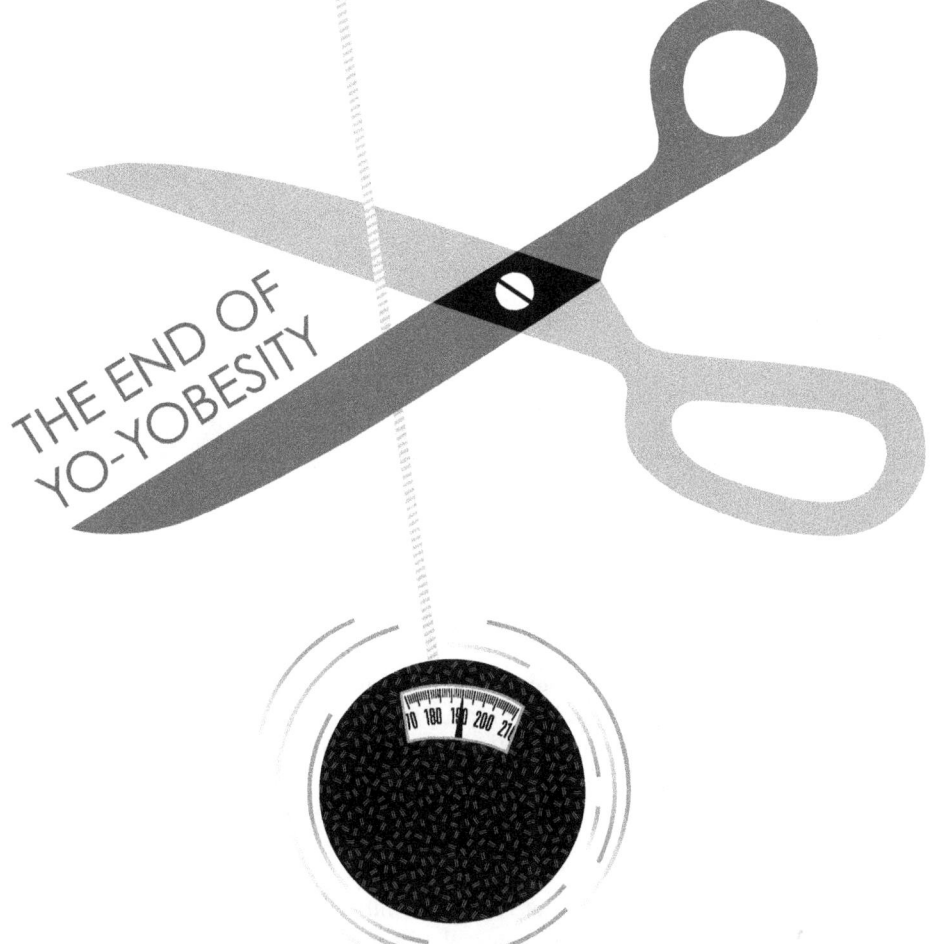

THE END OF YO-YOBESITY

TESSA WIZON

Resetting Normal: The End of Yo-yobesity
by Tessa Wizon
Published by New Perspectives Press
www.ResettingNormal.com

© 2018 Tessa Wizon

All rights reserved. No portion of this book may be reproduced in any form without permission from the publisher, except as permitted by U.S. copyright law. For permissions contact:

tessa@ResettingNormal.com

Cover art and book design by Kim Carney.
Illustrations by David Miller.
millercarneymiller.com

ISBN: 978-1-7321563-0-2 (paperback)
ISBN: 978-1-7321563-1-9 (digital)

FOR

Faye, John, Vanessa and Stephanie

ACKNOWLEDGEMENTS

Writing this book was a personal commitment that took far longer than I ever imagined. The ideas are from my personal experience, and the first draft was entirely a solo activity. However, transforming the manuscript from my first draft into final publication quality required expertise I didn't have. And I am grateful to the friends, professionals, and family members who helped me with that difficult task.

I'd like to thank my longtime friend Loretta Rippee, a hypnotherapist who works with clients wanting to lose weight, for reading two early versions of my manuscript and giving me detailed feedback that helped me improve the organization and make it more relevant for readers. I also thank her for her constant support and her patience in listening to some of my unorthodox ideas, judgement-free.

I'm grateful to Bonnie Goren, another longtime colleague and friend, for our enlightening discussions on the how and why of my approach to solving the weight problem. Challenging many of my convictions, she provided me with lots of practice explaining and defending them. She also read an early version of the book and gave me helpful feedback and support. And I'm extremely thankful she volunteered to test all my recipes, as I know from experience that she has in-depth culinary expertise.

Another very important person who helped me is Sandra Kersten Chalk. She was my first professional editor and she had quite a challenge guiding me in cutting my 560-page manuscript down to a readable length. I resisted every step of the way, but she persisted with patience and I am grateful for that. I also call her my Encourager in Chief. She believed in my message and at times when I wondered if my concept was worth publishing, she gave me hope that I did indeed have valuable information that could help other people.

I am immensely grateful to designer Kim Carney for the cover art that encapsulates the Yo-Yobesity concept and for the overall book design. And for illustrator David Miller for his fun graphics. I had a number of ideas for small graphics at various places in the text and Kim and David were able to take my vague descriptions and translate them into amusing images that help get my points across.

I would also like to acknowledge The Editorial Department (TED), a company that provides excellent manuscript editing services. Peter Gelfen advised me on content organization and Julie Miller did a thorough job copyediting my manuscript. I learned a lot about presenting ideas with clarity and about the mechanics of grammar – the book would not have been very professional without their help.

Regarding the endless, tedious tasks involved in actually getting a book published, I must thank Beth Jusino, a writer, developmental editor and publishing consultant who helped me navigate the confusing path to self-publishing. It isn't as easy as it looks, and her guidance was essential to my success.

Finally, I can't end without giving credit to my husband Phil, my kids Faye, John, and Vanessa, and my granddaughter Stephanie, as well as my brother Jerry and his wife Irene, who have listened to me talk about this project for more than a dozen years. They might not realize it, but their little suggestions dropped here and there along the way helped shape the final message. And Stephanie invented one of my favorite terms in the book, "snacktivity", which perfectly expresses the Western normal's habit of continuous snacking – I suspect (and hope) one day she'll become a writer. Thank you all.

TABLE OF CONTENTS

PART 1: INTRODUCTION
- Chapter 1: Who Should Read This Book? 7
- Chapter 2: Why Listen to Me? 10
- Chapter 3: How to Get the Most Out of This Book 12

PART 2: THE EXPERIMENT
- Chapter 4: My Story 13
- Chapter 5: Translating Experience Into a Plan 27
- Chapter 6: Resetting Normal – Overview 37

PART 3: THE PLAN
- Chapter 7: The Battle of the Mind 43
- Chapter 8: The Battle of Activity 70
- Chapter 9: The Battle of Quality 108
- Chapter 10: The Battle of Quantity 157
- Chapter 11: The Final Frontier 191
- Chapter 12: Tips for Keeping Your New Normal Forever 197

PART 4: SPECIAL CASES
- Chapter 13: How to Improve Quality on a Limited Budget 198
- Chapter 14 Resetting Normal for Kids 204

PART 5: WRAPPING IT UP
- APPENDIX A: WHOLE-FOOD ALTERNATIVES (RECIPES) 212
- APPENDIX B: ACTIONS TOOLS 231
- APPENDIX C: ADDITIVES AND PRESERVATIVES 243
- APPENDIX D: ADDITIONAL READING 245
- ENDNOTES 248
- INDEX 249

PART 1: INTRODUCTION
CHAPTER 1
WHO SHOULD READ THIS BOOK?

ASK YOURSELF: How many diets you have tried? If the answer is more than one, then you might be a yo-yo dieter—someone who cycles between denial/weight loss and indulgence/weight gain. Yo-yo dieting is the curse of the modern health quest. If one diet doesn't work we just blame ourselves for the failure and try another, eternally hopeful that we'll find one that does work. But the end result is gradual weight gain because with each cycle we invariably gain more than we lose. Welcome to yo-yobesity!

We endure a continual barrage of obesity warnings from all corners of the health industry. Experts want us to lose weight to get healthy, but they all advocate one primary solution—dieting. There's just one tiny problem: the success rate of this method has been dismal. People have been trying to lose weight by dieting for a century, at least. Yet the population at large is—well—just getting larger.

Today, you can assume almost every person in the country has been on a diet, is on one now, is trying to adhere to one, or thinks they should. Diet regimens have become billion-dollar businesses, and people have been dieting either by themselves or in some expensive diet program for well over fifty years.

But ask yourself the following questions:
- If so many people have been dieting in so many ways for so long, why is the obesity problem getting worse?
- If dieting were the answer, wouldn't it have solved the problem long ago? Wouldn't we all be svelte and fit and leaping around like deer in the forest?

Why don't diets work? It's because none of the experts can answer the following question: Even if you manage to lose weight on a diet (any diet), how do you maintain that for the rest of your life? Most diet programs profess to train you for maintenance, but all of them rely on self-control, willpower, and some level of denial. Who can tolerate that for a lifetime? Who even wants to?

What if I told you there's another way that's not a diet? A way that's not a diet but a transformation—a transformation that solves the problem so completely, you never need to think about dieting again. How would you feel if you never felt compelled to step on the scale again? If you never needed to track calories, fat grams, or carbs? If you never needed to count every step you take every day? If you never gained weight on vacations or holidays? And what if I told you that once you complete this transformation, you can eat whatever you want, whenever you want to?

Would you believe me? Probably not. And I would understand because I wouldn't believe it either if I hadn't gone through the transformation myself.

To get a glimpse into this future that awaits you, try to imagine a state in which you don't have to obsess about what and how much to eat, don't have to choose between guilt and deprivation, and don't have to start a diet every Monday or a whole new diet and exercise program every January 2nd. A state where you can channel all the energy formerly wasted on those efforts into what you *really* want to do with your life.

If you're a confirmed yo-yo dieter like I used to be, you probably can't. But that state is where I am *now*. And it could be where *you* are in the future. *Resetting Normal* will prove to you first that it's possible to achieve such a state, and second, how to do it yourself.

Resetting Normal is a permanent solution because anything normal is easy to maintain: you don't have to think about it, you just do it, without undue stress. For example, if it's normal for you to start your day with coffee, you just get up and make it or you pick it up on your way to work. You don't go through an agonizing decision every morning about whether to do it or not.

Consider: for most people, our current Western lifestyle is the norm. Unfortunately, this normal simply does not support good health or an optimally healthy weight for you. To improve your health, lose weight, and keep it off forever, what you need to do is change to a better normal. While that may sound impossible, you have the power to do it—*Resetting Normal* will show you how.

All it takes is winning four battles. Now, it might seem like fighting battles is an intimidating, negative approach to the problem. Who wants to fight? And why should you? But what is dieting? Dieting is a continual battle against yourself: what you want to eat vs. what you think you should eat. Weakness vs. willpower. Enjoyment vs. misery. How many win that battle? On the other hand, the battles to reset normal are winnable. You wage them not against yourself but against the outside influences that keep you trapped in a weight-gain cycle. You stop fighting yourself, you learn to leverage your own personal metabolism.

When you win these battles, you will reset your body to a new, healthier normal. Then you're done for life. You'll experience a sense of relief and freedom you never had before. No more dieting. Ever. You will win the prize: a totally natural, healthy, guilt-free relationship with food and activity that produces a normalized body weight.

Resetting Normal is for every one of you...
- Who doesn't feel you are as healthy as you could be
- Who hasn't had long-term success with any of the current diet plans
- Who's sick and tired of so-called experts telling you what, when, and how much to eat ... and then changing that recommendation every couple of weeks
- Who's sick and tired of those same experts telling you how much and when to exercise ... and then changing that recommendation every couple of weeks
- Who's sick and tired of being accused subtly and not so subtly of gluttony, stupidity, ignorance, and weak willpower
- Who has other goals in life besides trying to stick to a diet

Join me in *Resetting Normal*—put an end to yo-yobesity. Take the pledge: No mo' yo-yo!

CHAPTER 2
WHY LISTEN TO ME?

Resetting Normal is based on my personal experience—years of it. I've recently passed the seventy-year mark, and I was on the wrong end of the diet stick for forty-three years. I've been through all the societal diet cycles—low-calorie, low-carb, low-fat, high-carb—and back again. Some of them worked in the short-term. Some didn't work at all. None worked in the long-term.

My experience also includes lots of different roles, which gives me a unique perspective. I understand firsthand the demands and frustrations of everyday life that drive overeating. I've studied it from the inside (one of the people with the problem), as well as from the outside (studying the problem as a detached observer).

I've been an overweight child, pre-teen, teen, and adult. I've experienced the peer pressure in elementary school, junior high school, high school, and college. I've been an overweight spouse, an overweight parent, a parent with overweight children, a parent returned to school, and a grandparent. I've been a stay-at-home parent, a working single parent, self-employed, and an employee of various companies. I've been pre-menopausal, menopausal and post-menopausal. And in between being fat I've also been reasonably thin—not very often, but at least enough to know that it feels good.

I'm not an expert by scientific standards but that turns out to be an asset: after all, it was the experts who led me astray for all those overweight years. Once I stopped listening to them I was free to experiment, and I found a solution that changed my life more profoundly than I ever expected. A solution that gives me peace of mind knowing I'll be as healthy as I can possibly be and I'll *never* have a weight problem again. *Ever.*

In the coming chapters I frequently chastise these experts, so I want to be clear who I'm referring to. I've taken the liberty of adopting the definition set out by author David H. Freedman in the introduction to his book, WRONG: *Why Experts* Keep Failing Us—and How to Know When Not to Trust Them*[1]:

> ... when I say "expert," I'm mostly thinking of someone whom the mass media might quote as a credible authority on some topic—the sorts of people we're usually referring to when we say things like, "According to the experts ..." These are what I would call "mass" or "public" experts, people in a position to render opinions or findings that a large number of us might

hear about and choose to take into account in making decisions that could affect our lives.

There are many professionals in the field of nutrition and health who truly are experts and make significant contributions every day. The problem is that they do so quietly. Unfortunately, it's the loud voices that hijack media attention and influence health policies and medical advice—even if they're wrong.

I'm certainly not qualified to give anyone medical advice. But my life experience qualifies me to understand the problems overweight people deal with, and my success in conquering my own weight problems qualifies me to describe to you how I did it. I will never say, "If I can do it, anyone can." But I will say, "If I can do it, it's possible."

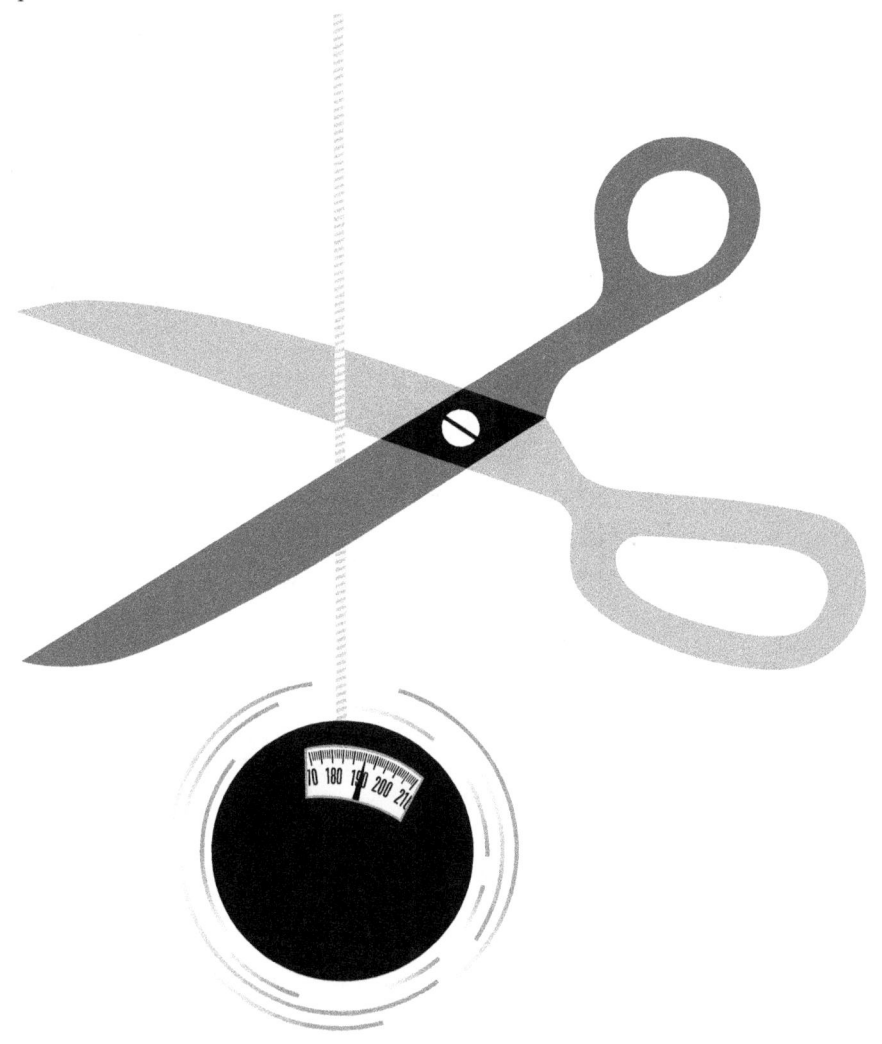

CHAPTER 3
HOW TO GET THE MOST OUT OF THIS BOOK

Resetting Normal contains everything you need to succeed in defeating yo-yo-besity: the background on how we got into this situation in the first place, how and why *Resetting Normal* works, the battle plans and the specific Actions for making it work for you. However, each person who has tried to lose weight and failed is an individual with a unique set of dietary experiences, likes and dislikes, and levels of dysfunction around eating, so I have also provided a corresponding workbook on the website **resettingnormal.com** where you can customize your experience.

The online workbook lists only the Actions, along with some extra detail and spaces for personal notes. You can download the workbook and either make your notes digitally on your favorite device or – if you prefer pen and paper – print out sections as needed and make your notes manually. That strategy allows you to choose which Actions are appropriate for you. Not everyone who wants to reset normal needs to complete all the Actions, as each of us comes from different lifestyle backgrounds. If you already practice some of the habits I recommend, you'll get through the program faster. But don't feel bad if you need to work on all the Actions—I certainly did.

I suggest you read all the way through the book first. Then go to the website and use the workbook to tackle the Actions you think you need to take. Some of those Actions are quick, mental exercises that only take a few minutes. Others will need to be repeated until you've absorbed them into your new normal.

PART 2: THE EXPERIMENT
CHAPTER 4
MY STORY

A history of dieting

If you have any kind of eating disorder (underweight, overweight, emotional eating or any other problem eating behavior), I understand you. I was one of you. Even if your problem is greater or lesser than mine, we share the same underlying problems and possibly the same solution. I suspect you will identify with most of the situations and feelings I describe below.

If you want the short list, here are a few of my stats:
- I was always chubby as a child.
- I came from a family where overeating was the norm.
- I started dieting at age twelve.
- I lived in a cycle of diet-on/diet-off.
- My adult height is five feet two.
- My weight at its highest point—excepting pregnancy—was 170 pounds.
- My weight when I quit dieting was 155 pounds.
- I am currently in my seventies.
- My current weight stays between 125 and 130 pounds (which I've maintained for more than ten years).

Today I count myself as one of those lucky people who sense when it's time to stop eating, but for most of my life that wasn't the case. I used to think it was genetic. Now I know it wasn't: I just developed some very bad eating habits as I grew up, and I carried them through most of my adult life.

GROWING UP WITH TMF (TOO MUCH FOOD)

I grew up in an era where the prevailing belief was that being "pleasantly plump" was healthy. My family always served a lot of good food—homemade and delicious, but it was a *lot* of food. And there was a subtle, underlying pressure to eat a lot.

It was also the clean-your-plate era. I don't criticize the *intent* of this principle—I certainly don't like to see people pile food on their plate and throw it away—and the immediate result was that I did always clean my plate. However, the unintended consequence of this policy was that instead of putting less on my plate so I could eat it all without getting stuffed, I just got used to eating more than I needed. In other words, the amount I put on my plate didn't shrink to fit my natural appetite; my appetite grew to accommodate the amount I put on my plate. And feeling stuffed became a normal feeling.

So it's no surprise I was an overweight child. I felt the effects by the time I was eight or nine years old. Just as it is today, those who weren't thin were excluded from the cool set, so my weight limited my social circle and lowered my self-esteem. It didn't help that some of kids nicknamed me "Tessie the dinosaur." By the time I was twelve—that age when the social scene becomes especially important—the weight thing really set in, and that's when I started dieting. After all, I'd need to be thin to attract the boys. And the quest to be a part of that thin group led to my series of diets.

You may recognize the cycle I went through for years.

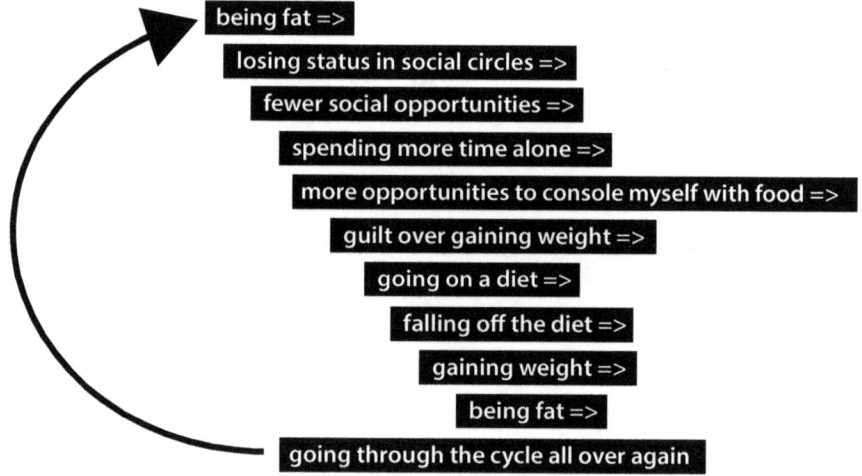

TEEN DIETS

Cottage cheese and peaches

My very first diet: eat cottage cheese and peaches three times a day for four days and lose five pounds. At age twelve I tried it and it worked. Of course, I gained it back in another couple of weeks, and for the next twenty years I didn't even want to *think* about cottage cheese and peaches.

Standard 1960s diet: low starch, low sugar, lean meat

In the 1960s the common belief was that too much starch, sugar, and fat was what made people fat, so going on a diet meant eating lean meats and limiting starches like potatoes, pasta, and desserts. For example, most family restaurants carried the a same typical diet plate: a lean hamburger patty (no bun), cottage cheese, lettuce and tomato, and a small cup of fruit. I tried this method for four months and it worked, too, but with the same long-term result—I gained it all back. Which didn't deter me from trying to do it over and over. Unfortunately, it got harder and harder until I finally gave up, destined to spend the rest of my teen years in the overweight category with a few close friends but no social life to speak of. I had entered early-stage yo-yobesity.

EARLY-ADULT DIETS

Post-college, during one of my low-weight periods, I did manage to socialize enough to develop a relationship and get married. But the ensuing motherhood generated additional pounds and the question of how to get rid of them again. Hope springs eternal, and just like most other people who diet, I blamed my previous failures to lose weight on myself while continuing to search for a diet that would work.

The Drinking Man's Diet: low-carbohydrate

My father had always fought a weight problem, too. He'd had success with a diet called *The Drinking Man's Diet*, created by Robert Cameron[2]. This diet took the approach that dieters could drink any amount of alcohol they wanted as long as it had no sugar in it. For example, bourbon with club soda was ok; wine and drinks made with sweet mixes were not. The diet allowed about fifty grams of carbohydrates per day, and dieters could eat as much protein and fat as they wanted. It wasn't nearly as severe in carbohydrate restriction as the Atkins Diet is, but it still didn't allow very much.

I tried it. I weighed about 160 pounds when I started. It took a lot of determination—life is full of carbs—but I stuck with the plan for six months and got my weight down to 115 pounds. I felt great! But once again, I couldn't stay there. After a few months, I was sick of protein overload, and cravings for the foods I hadn't let myself eat during the diet got the better of me. I gradually started gaining the weight back.

I went through this low-carb diet two more times over the following fifteen years. I could never hold onto the weight loss for more than six months and after a while I just got used to being a citizen of the Land of the Fat and Ugly: mid-stage yo-yobesity.

Maintaining a state of hunger + walking

At the ripe old age of thirty-nine—after fifteen years as a stay-at-home mom raising three kids, and three years into my second round of college—I didn't want to reenter the workforce in a year as a fat person. Determined to get the weight off no matter what, I cut back on everything. I ate what everyone else ate, just not very much of it. I was so busy with the kids, school, and working part-time it was easy to distract myself from food. As part of that distraction I also began my habit of walking—the one habit I gained during those years that has continued to benefit my health. I just started walking a little every morning, gradually working up to three miles.

I went hungry a lot of the time, regarding hunger as a signal that I was losing weight. And I did. I succeeded in losing about forty pounds, once more getting down to 115. But by now you know the story: I gradually gained most of the weight back.

DIETING BECOMES AN OBSESSION

Still, I was determined not to give up. I got serious with educating myself about nutrition and I began doing a lot of reading, investigating other kinds of diets. During the next decade I tried many of them—some with more success than others, but none that stabilized my weight. The most disturbing trend during this time was my growing obsession with food: what it consisted of, how I prepared it, and when and how much I was allowed to eat. On some of these diets I made everything from scratch myself, calculating the calories and fat in each serving, and I kept a diary of everything I ate every day, even adding up the total calories and fat at the end of each day and each week.

But there was an unintended consequence: I micro-managed my eating so much during the work week that when the weekend arrived I went crazy. Then the more I ate over the weekend, the more penitent I was on Monday, and the more restrictive I was Monday through Friday to try to compensate for the weekend binging ... which resulted in even more binging the following Saturday and Sunday. Sometimes I ate anything I could find until I was so full I couldn't eat any more—stuffed to the max. In one of those days I could consume more than 5000 calories. I know that number because in an effort to curb my binges (by shocking myself), I made myself write down everything I ate and add it up. It didn't work. It only succeeded in making me depressed and more determined to make up for it the following week. I had entered the advanced stage of yo-yobesity.

Just for the record, here are a few of the diets I tried during my advanced period.

The body-type diet

This diet assigned a body type to people based on their shape and metabolism, then laid out kinds of foods and eating schedules for each type. My particular type dictated that I eat very little for breakfast—only a little fruit. Then for lunch and dinner I could eat eggs, cheese, and rice, as well as unlimited amounts of some vegetables. I did lose some weight. But I couldn't handle the morning without any substantial food. By 11:00 a.m. I was counting the minutes until I could eat lunch. I felt like I was entering starvation mode—which I probably was. Eventually I fell back into the familiar pattern of restriction on weekdays and binging on the weekends, and after three months, gave it up altogether.

The very low-fat diet

During the late 1980s and early 1990s the low-fat, high-carb diet became a national trend. Susan Powter's book *Stop the Insanity!* [3] declared that dieting was insane. Her solution to fight dieting hunger was to consume lots of low-fat foods. Her theory: dieters who cut out the fat could up the quantity of everything else, feel full and still lose weight. In addition, she recommended a lot of exercise: she herself became a fitness instructor and claimed she could consume thousands of calories every day with her food and exercise regimen.

I gave it a try, sometimes getting my daily fat down below 10 percent. I made everything myself and kept track of all calorie and fat intake. But two things happened that made me quit. For one, after three months and no weight loss I realized I was never able to keep the calorie count low enough because the lack of fat kept me continually hungry and snacking on low-fat foods. Second, I began to have problems focusing my mind on anything—not a good thing when I was writing computer code—a symptom I later learned can be caused by too little fat in the diet. Since it wasn't working anyway, I abandoned it.

The Atkins Diet

Dr. Atkins' Diet Revolution[4] was relatively new at the time, similar to *The Drinking Man's Diet* but much more restrictive. So restrictive, in fact, that I lasted less than a week; my body is just not designed to handle that much protein and fat. The more protein I ate, the stronger my cravings for carbs became. By the third day I was ready to kill someone just for a grape. This diet definitely wasn't me.

Some whacko diet I read about in a magazine

I didn't usually take on what I considered whacko-type diets, but this one had me curious and I was getting desperate. Based on some theory about how the body processes carbohydrates, it maintained I could eat all the carbohydrates I wanted if I ate them at one meal and within one hour. That meant if I put up with only protein and fat for breakfast and lunch, I could eat potatoes, bread, cornbread, rice, pasta, cake, pie or whatever else with my dinner—as long as I consumed it within one hour. Who could resist? Not me, and I was astonished that it seemed to work. For two weeks I followed this eating pattern and I actually lost weight. I was ready to live with this diet forever! Then came the third week: no weight loss. Then the fourth week: weight gain. At that point I scratched it—I should've known it would be too good to be true. Of course it was a dumb thing to do, but I mention it because it shows how desperate we can get for diet solutions, no matter how ridiculous.

Finally, The Zone—the answer?

Then I heard about *The Zone Diet*[5]. I read the book and it seemed to be a reasonable approach based on rigorous scientific research. Advocating balancing everything we eat in certain proportions of protein, carbohydrate, and fat, it provided a simplified way of calculating what to eat and how to do that. The diet was balanced enough that my weekend binging subsided. So once again (and for the last time), over six months I got my weight down to 115. Of all the diets I've been on, this one was by far the most successful. I didn't maintain the 115 for more than a few months, but I did maintain my weight in the mid-120s for a couple of years—the longest I'd ever stabilized. I thought I'd found the answer.

There were some problems, however, that should have clued me in. I was still obsessed with preparing and tracking my food. I avoided eating out because it was impossible to choose a Zone-friendly meal at a restaurant. And there were some aspects of the food program I began to tire of: trying to make every eating encounter (meal or snack) in the correct Zone proportions annoyed me, and I didn't like having to add protein powder to cereals to properly balance them. Still, I thought I'd found the most reasonable solution available, and I thought if I ever started to gain weight again I'd have a fallback plan that wouldn't fail me. But not quite.

MAJOR LIFE TRANSITION

Menopause. I think menopause was the last straw. It's true that your metabolism declines at this point and unless you adjust your food intake, you'll put on weight. And I did. I tried valiantly to fix it with the Zone diet: I would dutifully start it every

Monday but could only stick with it three or four days before falling into binge mode. I'd lose five pounds, then gain six, lose three, gain five … gradually moving back up the scale. All the way back up to the low 150s. I wasn't happy about it, but nothing worked the way it used to. This was severe yo-yobesity syndrome at work.

THE TURNING POINT

The Zone had fizzled and it seemed the best I could do was to keep from gaining too much weight. It was depressing. I'd reached the end of my ability to deal with the situation using standard dieting methods. I just couldn't do it anymore.

So I gave up.

And that was the beginning of my success in solving the problem of a lifetime. It's also what this book is all about.

How I solved my weight problem

After the failures of The Zone—which had become exhausting and demoralizing—I finally admitted defeat. It was January 2001, and I said to myself, "What the [bleep] are you doing? Take a serious look at your life up till now: you keep doing the same thing over and over and failing over and over. You've been dieting since you were twelve years old. One diet after another. You've lost fifty pounds multiple times and each time gained it back. You lose ten pounds and you gain twelve. You lose five and you gain ten. You're fifty-five years old. You will never be the thin person you want to be; if you haven't done it by now, it just isn't going to happen. So accept your fate. Just stop the dieting and whatever happens, happens. It's time to throw in the towel."

Now, I want to emphasize that this was a *huge* capitulation for me.

First of all, I've never been one to give up on something I wanted to do. Second, I had an extreme fear of what would happen if I stopped controlling my diet.

I'd always believed that my metabolism was broken. I believed I would always eat more than I needed (because I always had), that I was always a little hungrier than I needed to be, and that if I didn't control that behavior, I'd gradually and continually gain weight until I became one of those people who weigh a thousand pounds and have to be removed from their house with a forklift. This is not an exaggeration. I seriously believed that about myself.

So, giving up that control took a *giant leap of faith*. I was just hoping against hope that my worst fears would not be realized. As a backup, I assured myself that if my new plan started to go terribly wrong I could always go back into control-freak mode. But I vowed to do that only as a last resort.

TAKING STOCK

Before I started, I took an assessment of what I was doing right and what I was doing wrong. On the plus side, I enjoyed cooking from scratch and I ate only a moderate amount of processed foods; I didn't drink soda; I'd been exercising pretty regularly since I was forty (walking and aerobics); my alcohol consumption was moderate. On the minus side, I had a weakness for homemade goodies (cookies, pie, pastry, specialty breads, and the like); I could eat my weight in noodles and potatoes; I was easily tempted by treats offered by others, like donuts; and I could eat way too much, especially when I was upset about other things in my life.

I concluded that my nemeses were cravings for the wrong kinds of foods, emotional eating habits, and eating too much overall. And dieting had fixed none of these problems.

THE PHASES AS THEY UNFOLDED

Phase I: Setting the Stage

Where to start? I wasn't sure—this was uncharted territory for me—but it didn't take long for me to realize I'd been dieting for so long I couldn't just stop cold turkey. I'd established many control mechanisms, including weighing myself every day and counting all kinds of food values. To stop my control cycle, I had to stop those behaviors. The first step I took was to hide some things. I put the scale in the garage where I couldn't easily get to it. I put my food-value reference books in an inaccessible box as well. The latter was a little less effective since I'd memorized most of them, but getting them out of my sight reminded me I should stop thinking about food that way.

Mentally, I encouraged myself to accept whatever happened.

Phase II: Deprogramming

With the arbitrary measuring tools out of the way, I set about deprogramming my diet mentality. This was *not* a trivial process. After forty-three years of dieting, that mentality had become so ingrained that I didn't eat anything without evaluating calories, fat, or carb values. I had to figure out a way to break this pattern. So I did the following:

- I gave myself permission to eat whatever I wanted, whenever I wanted, just *not in unlimited quantities*.
- I fought the clear-the-deck mentality—eating all the forbidden goodies on Sunday so as not to be tempted on Monday—by making myself eat them a little at a time throughout the following week.

The surprising result. At face value, this approach seems like it should've been a disaster. But amazingly, *the feared weight gain never materialized.* As a matter of fact, *within two months* I'd achieved something I'd never thought possible. My eating patterns leveled out. I no longer binged on the weekends. *I had broken the insidious pattern of denial and indulgence.* And while I wasn't weighing myself, I knew that I hadn't gained weight because my clothes fit the same. It was my first successful blow against yo-yobesity.

A powerful discovery. As time progressed and I adjusted to the diet-free mentality, I made a powerful discovery: when I allowed myself to eat whatever I wanted whenever I wanted, I became *more and more selective* about both of those options. I began to ask myself:

- Do I really want *this* food?
- Do I want this food *now*?

And surprisingly, sometimes the answer was no. I'd ask myself, "If I can have this [donut/muffin/cookie/candy/pizza ...] now or an hour from now or tomorrow, when would I prefer to eat it?" Or looking at the flip side, "Since I can have this anytime I want, I don't have to eat it all now. I can have one small piece now and if I want more an hour from now, I can have more." What shocked me was that as time went on, I became more inclined to eat that first small piece and wait. Frequently, I found that later I didn't want more, or I'd get busy with work and forget about it. That had *never* happened to me before. In the past I was always, always thinking about food—what I was going to eat and how long until I was allowed to eat it. And believe me, I would never have passed up an opportunity to scarf something down if I had the chance.

The beginning of the transformation. I expanded my self-questioning to include, "If you could choose any food you wanted for this meal, what would it be?" And that simple question began to put me in touch with my body's nutritional and metabolic requirements. When I listened to my body's answer to that question and ate accordingly, I felt satisfied and didn't need to think about eating for a long time. I learned that hunger is driven by lack of satisfaction and has little to do with physical fullness. Eating a plateful of cauliflower didn't give me satisfaction if my body was asking for was cheese.

As I became more practiced at this, my obsession with food lessened. I could eat and then forget about food until my stomach reminded me I was hungry, which could be hours later. And as an added benefit, losing my obsession with food allowed me to focus on other things I wanted to accomplish in my life. I was more productive at work, no longer experiencing periods of time when I was so hungry I couldn't think about anything else.

Phase III: Making some adjustments

Taking stock again. The goal up to this point had been to stop gaining weight, get dieting out of my head, and get the concept of forbidden foods out of my head. I was about 60 percent of the way there and my weight was stable in a way it had never been in my entire life.

However ... a part of me had hoped I might *lose* a little weight in the process, and I hadn't. Time to make some adjustments. But how to make adjustments that might result in weight loss without going back to dieting? I had to come to terms with the fact that some foods—like pastries, desserts, and candy—aren't good for anyone in large quantities, even if they're homemade. Problem was, I liked them and didn't want to give them up entirely. I decided on a compromise. I tried two experiments.

Trial one: crowding out the goodies. This meant eating the whole foods first. For example, if I wanted a donut in the morning I had eggs first. The protein and fat from the eggs filled me up and helped me limit the donut consumption to a small piece. It was a win-win because I still got to have a little of the donut experience. Another example: if I wanted a cookie for dessert, I ate some fruit first. These were indeed small changes, but the result over time was that I began to prefer this way of eating. It didn't feel like denial because I wasn't eliminating these foods entirely, just eating a little less.

Trial two: experimenting with quantity. Allowing myself to eat anything I wanted had produced good results in eliminating the yo-yo eating behavior, but frequently I still ate too much and felt stuffed afterward. (It was rare for me to undereat.) I came up with the idea of a post-meal evaluation. I tried to remember approximately how much I ate and then one hour later ask myself how I felt: still hungry, stuffed, or just right? If I was still hungry I'd eat more next time, and if I felt stuffed I'd eat less. I was aiming to eventually hit *just-right* most of the time.

This process took considerable experimentation. I instinctively knew it was important to physically feel the just-right state, but I rarely could and that frustrated me. At the time I tried to be happy for whatever success I could achieve.

The continuation of the surprising results. Week by week, asking myself the feedback questions, it was getting easier to eat the new way.

The continuation of the transformation. The fact that I was beginning to prefer fewer sweets and starchy foods could only mean one thing: *my tastes were changing.* What wouldn't have satisfied me before was now quite satisfying. Many of my former cravings had just disappeared. A diet requiring me to suddenly stop eating these foods wouldn't have accomplished the same thing. My body was responding to the gradual changes by sending me comforting signals and thus encouraging me to continue.

Phase IV: Adding exercise

Taking stock again. So far so good. I felt like I was eating in a healthier way, cutting back on the sweet stuff and the snacks. I wasn't gaining weight and had even shrunk a little.

However ... I'd hoped the tweaks I implemented would cause me to lose a little *more* weight, and that still hadn't happened. My clothes felt an itty-bit looser but not much.

Was exercise the missing key? I'd been exercising fairly regularly since I was thirty-nine when I lived in Southern California, with walking and aerobics in the morning before work. However, after moving to Seattle, with its long periods of darkness, I'd slacked off. Joining a gym seemed to be the only other option even though it meant getting up super early in the morning. At the gym I learned some moderate weight lifting techniques. And after some experimentation, I finally settled on a weight workout twice a week and a cardio workout the remaining three.

The surprising results. It didn't take long for me to feel the benefits. My stamina increased. I stood taller. The fat I was carrying shifted to better places. I felt fit. I continued to maintain the eating patterns I'd established. But *I was still not getting much thinner.* Maybe a little, but not enough to notice. It was an aaarrrrgh! moment.

Phase V: Finally losing weight

Taking stock again. Regardless, I chose to be happy with my results to date; I didn't let my lack of weight loss discourage me. Since I was doing this on my own, there was no one (diet book or diet expert) to tell me I was a failure. Just maintaining a stable weight was a *huge* reward in itself. By this time my diet consisted mostly of healthy food, and the exercise had really boosted my level of fitness and energy.

Continuing the tweaks. I continued to build on the tweaks I'd added earlier. Expanding the crowding-out techniques became easier every week. I still ate whatever I wanted, whenever I wanted, but the fewer pastries, cookies, and so on that I ate, the less I desired them. There were times when someone brought goodies to work and I found I didn't want any. This was a surprising and empowering experience.

Quantity—the final frontier. All this left one eating behavior I hadn't yet conquered: *how much* to eat. I was still eating too much. It was just hard to reconcile what I saw on my plate with what would fill me up. Perception is so powerful; even knowing the overstuffed feeling from experience, I couldn't always control it.

I had to find a way to fight my long-held perceptions about what an appropriate quantity of food for me actually looks like. Most of us who have a weight problem are dependent on outside influences to determine how much to eat. As children we learned it from parents or other adult role models. Then as adults, experts and social norms take the place of parents. We never learned to listen to our own built-in *appestat*—appetite regulator.

It turns out that resetting my perception of a normal quantity was the hardest thing to do. Building on my just-right technique was just the beginning. I had to figure out how to dislodge my old perceptions and replace them with new ones. Over time I devised techniques to help me block out outside influences and reactivate my appestat. Once my appestat took control, eating an appropriate, satisfying quantity was no longer a problem. Then, with a few minor tweaks, my weight dropped to where I wanted it to be.

The state of my transformation. I finally achieved my primary goals. I stopped my yo-yo dieting. I reduced my consumption of junk foods by replacing them with healthy whole foods I liked. I became more fit by exercising regularly. And finally, I'd lost some weight.

Each phase was crucial in my transformation. It might look like the last thing I tried—reducing quantity—was the real solution. Couldn't I have just done that in the first place? But I'd already tried that with other diets, and I'd always failed. *I never could have gotten to that last step without going through the others first. My success lay in compounding all the changes I implemented from the start.*

Phase VI: Testing it

Ok—I felt I'd arrived. But was this for real? Was this permanent? I'd landed at my ideal size, and I continued to eat the new way I'd become used to. Over time my size and my weight remained stable. I never weighed myself at home, but through weigh-ins at my doctor's visits, I knew it stayed the same.

After two years of this stability I decided it was a done deal. I had defeated yo-yobesity! No mo' yo-yo!

The end result

My end result is better than ever I could have imagined: I've created a new normal for me. *The final transformation changed my relationship to food and therefore changed my life.* I never think about my weight. I never think about going on a diet. I don't count calories or carbs or fat grams or anything else. I don't crave, agonize, or obsess about food. I don't gain weight on weekends. I don't gain weight on vacations. I don't gain weight over the holidays. Yes, I do eat holiday goodies—just not tons of them—but when January rolls around and everyone else is making diet and exercise resolutions, I just go back to my new normal. Even if I've put on a few pounds they disappear in no time, with no additional effort on my part. I eat what I want, choosing from a vast array of real foods, based on my preferences in the moment. I have become one of those people I always used to envy: those who know when they're full and are able to happily stop eating at that point.

I *didn't just win the battle, I won the war.* There is no more fighting with myself. No "I wish I could have that but I can't because I'm on a diet." I have a huge palette of foods to choose from—all of which I really like and all of which are good for me, even an occasional high-quality dessert (yes, real cheesecake isn't going to kill you if you don't eat it every day). The food I eat is satisfying and I only eat what I need to fill up, not to stuff myself into oblivion. I no longer carry the one-hundred-pound load of diet thinking on my shoulders. The stress of always exerting control over my eating is gone. The stress of thinking about the next diet is gone. Eating has become a natural, enjoyable part of my life and my health is good. In a few words, my new way of eating has become my normal and because of that, it's maintenance free. Yo-yobesity is a thing of the past.

WHAT I LEARNED

My dietary experience taught me a real lesson: if you've tried and tried again and still failed, maybe you set the wrong goal. I was trying and trying to lose weight by dieting, measuring progress in pounds lost and failing time after time. Then, when I finally took my focus off counting lost pounds and put it on what and how I ate, I did lose weight *as a side effect.*

I was totally unprepared for where my changes would take me in the long run. Most of my life I'd been forcing and forcing and forcing—pounding the square peg into the round hole—because that's what I thought I should do. Then, when I stopped, when I let go of those old precepts, it was like a *Star Trek* worm hole had opened up in the time-space continuum and I went straight to where I wanted to go. For me, my whole food world changed.

THERE IS NO SHORT-CUT, BUT ...

It took me almost four years to achieve the final results I was looking for. But don't assume it will take you that long. It took me only two months to lay the foundation for success: stopping the yo-yo diet behavior in its tracks and ending weight gain. The rest of the time was spent in a process of experimentation because what I was attempting to do went against everything I'd read and heard in the last fifty years about nutrition and losing weight. I had to figure things out as I went, which included many failures along the way to success. In *Resetting Normal* I have handpicked what worked so you don't have to waste time going down unproductive paths.

Yes, there is no short cut to permanent weight loss. But spending the rest of your life on one diet after another will take far longer than resetting your normal just once.

NOTES

CHAPTER 5
TRANSLATING EXPERIENCE INTO A PLAN

Origin

As you can see, I didn't start out with the idea of *resetting normal*. There was no master plan and no particular goal. Only one thing was clear to me: I knew I couldn't keep on with the dieting paradigm I'd been following for most of my life. I started on my journey and followed it wherever it took me. I tried many different approaches. If something worked I kept doing it. If it didn't work I stopped doing it. And somehow, through all those trials I found the sweet spot—a solution to the Big Question of our time: How can we stop obesity in its tracks?

My personal success is so complete I think it's worth sharing—I'm certainly not the only person on the planet with a weight problem. Even if my solution doesn't work for everyone, it can't have a more dismal success rate than what the current experts are selling. But to share my success I had to look back over everything I did, separate what worked from what failed, and organize it into a plan with steps that someone else could easily follow.

The concept of *resetting normal* came out of that retrospective thinking—a realization that everything I changed gradually over time became normal for me and consequently stable. And that explains why it's so effortless to maintain.

FRAMING THE REAL PROBLEM

Health experts in our country have created such an intense obsession over the effect of weight on health, we have the impression that thin = healthy. This assumption is false; while you *can* be thin and healthy, *thinness doesn't guarantee health*. Unfortunately, it leads to the belief that weight itself is the primary problem and you can't get healthy without fixing the weight first.

Through the process of *resetting normal*, I discovered that this traditional approach is backwards. When you're overweight (or underweight, for that matter), your internal metabolism is so out of whack it gives you all the wrong appetite signals, making self-control hard, succumbing to temptation easy, and adhering to a diet nearly impossible. Those conditions make it extremely difficult to fix the weight problem first, and if you can't do that, according to this paradigm, you can never even get to the health issue. Wrong problem, wrong solution. *Resetting Normal* reverses that approach. You don't lose weight to get healthy, *you get healthy and then lose weight*.

I like metaphors, and the following joke by Jerry H. Simpson, Jr., from *Reader's Digest: Laughter, The Best Medicine*[6] expresses this idea perfectly:

> *The zoo built a special eight-foot-high enclosure for its newly acquired kangaroo, but the next morning the animal was found hopping around outside. The height of the fence was increased to 15 feet, but the kangaroo got out again. Exasperated, the zoo director had the height increased to 30 feet, but the kangaroo still escaped. A giraffe asked the kangaroo, "How high do you think they'll build the fence?"*
>
> *I don't know, said the kangaroo. "Maybe a thousand feet if they keep leaving the gate unlocked."*

Just like the zookeeper, we've been focused on the wrong thing. The zookeeper sees only the fence and totally misses the gate. We see only weight—the symptom—and completely overlook the real causes—the internal and external factors that drive weight gain. *Resetting Normal* identifies those factors and provides the tools to fix them. Health first, weight second.

The metaphor for *Resetting Normal*

I use the terms "battle" and "war" to explain the process and there's a reason for that: we are surrounded by environmental forces that drive our unhealthy normal. There are those who like to point to someone they think looks overweight and claim, "It's your own fault you're fat! Ipso fatso, just control yourself!" But it's not that simple. In the last century, forces in our Western environment have created a perfect obesogenic storm and we're caught in the middle. The only way to survive it is to fight our way out of it and fortify our defenses against it for the future.

According to an article published in *The Lancet*, Boyd Swinburn[7], a medical researcher working for the NIH and studying the severe obesity and health problems of the Pima Indians in Arizona in the late 1980s, concluded that "obesity was just a normal physiological response to an abnormal environment." Later he coined "obesogenic" as the term for this environment.

Much of the research today is focused on identifying potential *internal* causes of obesity: genetics, hormones, addictions, fat metabolism, and so on. I'm sure these factors have an influence, but my personal experience has me agreeing with Swinburn—the primary culprit is the forces in our environment. We can't change that environment, but we can fight against it and win at a personal level.

The forces we must fight

OUR WESTERN NORMAL

What is the Western normal?

Our Western normal is a huge problem for us. Consider both our food supply and our lifestyle.

Food. The normal food in our culture does not support good health. Most of the foods available in stores are convenience-based: highly processed, cheap, and available anytime, night or day. Processed food is what people think of as normal and we have labelled people who try to eat better as "health nuts." Not eating cheeseburgers, French fries, pizza, and Oreos somehow seems un-American.

Lifestyle. The normal Western lifestyle doesn't support good health either. It doesn't lend itself to physical activity. Too many of us have desk jobs and long commutes. Many of us are expected to work long hours, take little time off, and stay connected via cell phone when not at work. Society also expects that we keep up with popular entertainment and participate in social media, and it's easy to sit in front of some electronic device until all hours of the night to fulfill that expectation. It's also easy to avoid daily physical activity because almost everything is automated: with microwave meals, dishwashers, washing machines, elevators, and even car-door openers, it's possible to go through an entire day with barely any physical effort.

What is the fight?

Most of us desire to be considered normal—at least in most ways. Human beings are social creatures, and it's built into our psyche to want to be part of the group. That makes it easy to go along with whatever everyone else is doing and hard to do something different. The Western normal—both food and lifestyle—does not support good health. If you want to improve your health, you must fight against that normal.

THE AGRICULTURE AND FOOD INDUSTRIES

Conflicting goals

Make no mistake: while *your* goal might be to live a long and healthy life, the goal of large-scale agriculture and food conglomerates is to make a profit. That means keeping production costs low, producing products that have a high profit margin, and marketing them aggressively, all regardless of their effects on our health. The result: highly processed foods. Over decades, the food industry has learned how to put a healthy spin on these products to trick consumers into thinking a product is healthy even if it's not.

And while a hundred years ago, most people ate three meals a day—they had no access to food in between—the food industry has made snacking and 24/7 food availability a major part of their marketing plan. They make sure food is within our grasp anytime, night or day, consequently making it normal for us eat all the time. And we do.

What is the fight?

The fight is to learn to distinguish between products that truly support health and those that sabotage it. It's to personally experience that whole, quality foods taste great. It's to eat foods that satisfy so you only want to eat when you're hungry—not just because food is within reach. And it's to acquire an arsenal of tools to defend yourself against the food industry's massive Marketing Machine.

A DIET-OBSESSED CULTURE

Why we are diet-obsessed

Considering that dieting fails for most of us, whether short-term or long-term, it's legitimate to ask why we still try to lose weight by dieting. The answer is twofold. First, the desire to be thin, whether for medical reasons or just to meet cultural expectations, forces us to keep at it. Books have been written on why the desire to become thin has taken over our psyche at the expense of almost every other aspect of our lives. And second, no one has come up with a workable alternative. Unfortunately, dieting creates a net negative for us across the board: it breeds unhealthy eating patterns, including eating disorders, and it keeps us from achieving the end goal of weight loss. Dieting not only doesn't work but is inherently destructive.

What is the fight?

The fight is growing the confidence to block out the onslaught of diet edicts from various public and private health experts, well-meaning relatives and friends, and thousands of diet books and websites, and empowering your own internal appestat to govern what and how much you eat.

A HISTORY OF BAD ADVICE

What bad advice?

Let's see: public and private health agencies have been hard at work modifying our behavior since the mid-twentieth century, yet we've arrived at a crisis with a so-called obesity epidemic and out-of-control medical costs. If all their advice has been on target, we shouldn't be in this position. They claim, naturally, that the reason there's a problem is that most people are not taking their advice, but that's not true. When the health agencies advised us to eat less butter, people switched to margarine. When they advised us to eat fewer eggs, egg consumption dropped so precipitously that egg farmers had to launch a counter campaign in order not to go out of business. When they advised us to eat low-fat and high-carb, people switched to low- or non fat products and ramped up consumption of bagels and pasta. And these are just a few of dozens of well-intentioned but disastrous pieces of advice the "experts" doled out.

Confronted with the results of their bad advice, these agencies respond with the equivalent of, "But that's not what we meant! When we said to eat fewer eggs, we really thought they were bad for you. When we said to eat low-fat, high-carb, we didn't mean replace the fat with refined carbohydrates like sugar and white flour products, we meant for you to replace them with vegetables, fruits, and whole grains. When we said to eat less butter, we didn't mean eat more margarine instead. And we didn't know how bad trans-fats were back then." The latter denial regarding trans-fats is not true—some scientists and nutritionists did know. Nutritionist Adelle Davis warned of the dangers in 1954 in *Let's Eat Right to Keep Fit:* "When fats are hydrogenated ... their health-building value is destroyed. Such fats can supply calories but nothing more ... neither can they support life of bug or beast."

The experts' track record doesn't exactly inspire my confidence in them. Unfortunately, it turns out that when you try to herd people in a different direction, the law of unintended consequences dictates that you don't necessarily have control over what their new direction will be. When you oversimplify to the point of reducing advice to marketable sound bites you leave out a lot of important information, and that leaves people to interpret your advice and follow it as best they can. And people did.

What is the fight?

Much like building a defense against food-industry marketing, we need to build a fortress against bad advice from well-meaning but frequently misguided health agencies. Go back to the basics, see the big picture, and stop trying to micromanage your body according the latest trendy health study. Learn to trust your own body and your own judgment. Reactivate your own internal appestat.

AN INSATIABLE MASS MEDIA
How the media influences us

"The media" or "mass media" can be defined as the means of communication that reaches large numbers of people. In our technologically driven age, this information is beamed at us twenty-four hours every day, creating a tsunami of edicts telling us what to do, what to eat, and how to live. That's why it has a tremendous influence on our health.

A mouthpiece. The media cover all kinds of health advice, both good and bad. That, in itself, is not detrimental. However, it also provides so-called experts a mouthpiece for questionable advice, misleading the average consumer who has neither the time nor the expertise to evaluate it.

Dumbing it down. Any scientist will tell you that the science of health is relatively incomplete because it is enormously complex. There is no such thing as a simple study. But the media are under pressure to report whatever it thinks will pique consumers' interest, and they have to do so in a short news brief, no matter how complex the concepts. The result: they dumb it down to bullet points. This oversimplification of a complex subject can only lead consumers into making behavioral changes which may not be in their best interest.

Creating an illusion of truth. Say something often enough and people will believe it's true. Repetition creates the *illusion of truth*. The media have plenty of bandwidth for repetition, which brainwashes consumers with incomplete information that may be detrimental to their health.

Too much study-driven health news. To get more eyeballs on their coverage, the media scour medical journals for studies with the most potential for sensational headlines. But studies are tools for scientists—they're steps along the way to truth, rarely conclusive—and it's all too easy to be misled into making self-treatment decisions based on partial information.

Shaping our concepts of a culturally acceptable body image. Until about a hundred years ago, our body image was shaped mostly by our local community: family, friends, and acquaintances. Not anymore. Today we have global coverage and technology. We live in an increasingly visual society, and our definition of beauty is shaped by digital cameras and software that can erase any imperfection and enhance any feature. So now, both men and women are constantly trying to live up to standards that aren't only unrealistic, they're impossible. This situation does not lead to good health. It leads to fad dieting, depression, and eating disorders.

Giving consumers mixed messages. Actually, the media present us with not just mixed messages, but conflicting messages. One says "Eat!" and the other says "Don't eat!" A magazine might feature an article about how to lose ten pounds in a week juxtaposed with a recipe for a triple chocolate cake. It's that denial-indulgence cycle rearing its ugly head again. Eat … don't eat, eat … don't eat, eat … don't eat … it's enough to drive you crazy!

An outlet for marketing so-called health products and medications. The increased interest in diet products, other health products, and medications means plenty of opportunities for the billion-dollar diet industry, the pharmaceutical industry, and the healthcare industry. The standards for such ads are so loose that many of them are misleading and some are outright fraud.

Promoting weight loss as entertainment. I understand that many people watched the show *The Biggest Loser* when it was on the air. And I'm sure the people who participated were hopeful this kind of exposure and pressure would help (force) them to lose weight. But I can't help but feel sad that so many people are so desperate, they'd subject themselves to such radical and humiliating circumstances. I'm happy for those few who succeeded, but presenting the show's model as a solution to a serious problem is more damaging than helpful because it isn't practical for the average person. Plus, a new study done in 2016[8] about what happens to the participants afterward shows that this severe approach to weight loss backfires, causing a host of metabolic side-effects. Shows like this are entertainment only.

What is the fight?

We must fight the continuous barrage of information with a healthy skepticism. We must learn how to distinguish fact from fiction and fact from fraud. We must fight the illusion of truth through repetition and resist marketing messages that aren't in our best interest.

"WE HAVE MET THE ENEMY … "

Who is the enemy?

"We have met the enemy and he is us."

In case you aren't old enough to remember *Pogo*, it was a satirical comic created by Walt Kelly[9] in the 1950s. Pogo was a possum living in the Okefenokee Swamp in a community of animal and reptile friends, engaging in adventures reflecting current human situations of the time. The title for this section quotes Kelly's 1971 Earth Day poster, which clearly illustrated that the escalating pollution of the environment is every individual's responsibility. There's a parallel here: in the current health crisis concerning weight, there is ample blame to be shared by the food industry, health agencies, the news media, and other segments of our society. But we also need to examine our own complicity. Here are some of the ways we all contribute to the problem.

We have forgotten that we are what we eat. What we eat is important for our health, but through other influences we have come to accept the Western diet of processed foods as normal and we don't think about what we're eating.

We love convenience. Our Western lifestyle fills our time completely, and it doesn't usually include time for planning, preparing, and consuming healthy whole foods. We may know we need to make the time, yet we are reluctant to make it a priority.

Selective rationalization—we pick and choose what is most convenient to believe. There is a ton of evidence now that processed foods simply don't make a good substitute for whole foods. But a lot of people just don't believe it or, more likely, *don't want* to believe it. Probably the real reason is that they've always eaten processed foods, enjoy them, and don't want to give them up, regardless of the evidence.

We like the idea of silver bullets. Everything in life is complex under the surface and it's hard to deal with, so it's not surprising that we long for simple solutions. Whether it's antioxidants, vitamin D, juicing, green tea, or some other elixir with the promise of long life, we want to believe it will work. And it's easier to take a couple of pills than to fix a real dinner.

We push the limits because we're used to medical miracles. We have an amazing medical system that performs medical miracles daily. Unfortunately, that has bred an expectation that our physicians and medicines should be able to fix everything. And *that* has led many to put prevention on the back burner because they feel that whatever goes wrong with their health, they can just take some pill or have an operation to fix it. Many people just don't get that it's a whole lot easier to prevent disease than to fix it later.

What is the fight?

Pogo was right. He was right about the environment, and he provided us with a truism that applies to our own health conundrum today. There's plenty of blame for things we have no control over, but we can't ignore our own responsibility. If we don't recognize that we are what we eat (literally), if convenience is our top priority, if we insist on believing that processed foods are just as good as the real thing, if we succumb to the allure of silver bullets, if we refuse to realize we need to change, and if we expect drugs and surgery to save us, then "We have met the enemy and he is us." We must win the battle against ourselves.

THE CONVERGENCE

Taken together, we're surrounded by armies of considerable force:
- What's normal in our society
- The profit motive and power behind all the industries around food and health
- Bad advice from experts
- A diet-obsessed culture
- An insatiable mass media that doesn't distinguish between information and misinformation
- Our own inclinations

I use the metaphor of a battle plan for *Resetting Normal* because the only way to win the war on weight is to win the battles against these forces.

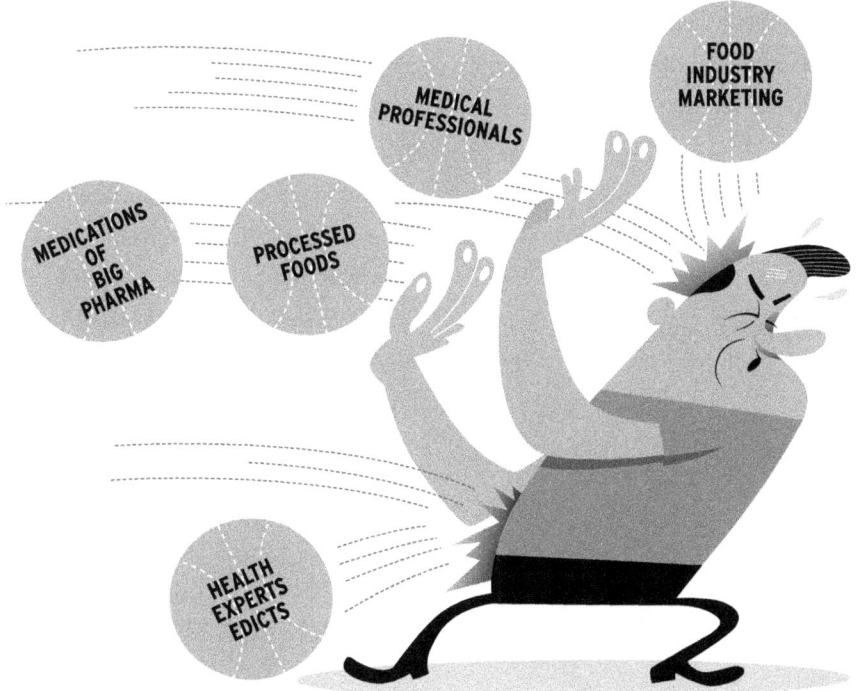

A permanent solution

Despite all the research and medical and public efforts to get people thinner, the experts have not been able to solve the following problem:

Even if you somehow manage to lose weight on a diet (any diet), how do you make the new, healthier way of eating and exercise last for the rest of your life?

You can pick just about any diet out there and if you follow the rules exactly, lose weight. Lots of people do that, over and over. There are countless methods and studies (many of them conflicting) about the best way to do it. Losing the weight is the easy part. *The real challenge is making the changes permanent.*

My way of *resetting normal* does just that.

Diet methods to date require you to step outside your normal and do something extraordinary. In our driven Western culture, the typically accepted view is that one has to set a goal and work like hell to achieve it. We see this approach as somehow morally superior—if you succeed you've put yourself to the test and passed. It's popular to liken our goals to climbing a mountain, running a marathon, or clawing our way up the corporate ladder. But there is *one huge flaw* in applying that kind of thinking to losing weight and getting healthier. When you have climbed that mountain or run that marathon, you claim your victory and then you're done. You don't have to keep doing it every day for the rest of your life. Losing weight and getting healthy need to last a lifetime, and treating them like a marathon makes them unsustainable.

The ultimate goal of this book's plan is to change your normal to one that is healthier. It's designed to take you step by step from your current normal to a new, healthier one whether you need to lose weight or not. The key to success is to get completely comfortable with each change before moving on to the next one. Don't try to rush your progress. You need to internalize each change and make it normal for you, or later you'll slide back to your old, familiar ways. Once you have completely adopted the new, healthier normal, *it becomes effortless to maintain.*

NOTES

CHAPTER 6
RESETTING NORMAL—OVERVIEW

The overall plan is not complicated. I've taken my experience and condensed the fights above into an easy-to-follow battle plan. To reset normal, you do have to wage this war and that may sound harsh. But in fact, it's a lot easier to fight back against outside influences than it is to fight with yourself (as you do when you diet). Here are the four battles you'll to need to tackle:

1) The Battle of the Mind
2) The Battle of Activity
3) The Battle of Quality
4) The Battle of Quantity

THE BATTLE OF THE MIND

To be successful *resetting normal* you need to adopt a new way of looking at the health/weight problem. The end goal is the same, but the path and timeline are different.

Goals:
- Create an environment that supports your new approach.
- Diet-proof yourself—stop the denial-indulgence cycle that drives yo-yobesity.
- Master the tools to make you expert-proof, social-proof, and commercial-proof.

THE BATTLE OF ACTIVITY

One thing that the experts are right about is that to be healthy, you need to engage in some kind of physical activity. However, you need to stop associating exercise solely with weight loss.

Goals:
- Recognize the benefits of physical activity.
- Stop measuring the success of exercise by weight loss.
- Learn simple ways to ramp up your everyday activity.
- Start engaging in some kind of physical activity to build endurance.
- Start engaging in some kind of physical activity to build strength.
- Understand the value of sleep.

THE BATTLE OF QUALITY

What you eat matters. Eating some processed foods will not harm you, but you put your health and your weight at risk if you eat a steady diet of them. Whole foods will fill you up *and* satisfy you (those two things are not the same), while processed foods will compel you to eat more. But the goal does not have to be a 100 percent whole-foods diet. I firmly believe in an 80/20 principle: if 80 percent of what you eat is good for you, the other 20 percent is not going to kill you. This battle is not about losing weight: it's about healing and restoration. In this battle you'll learn how to use RESET (**R**esearch; **E**xperiment; **S**ubstitute; **E**valuate; **T**est) to find food replacements you *like*.

Goals:
- Learn how to identify processed foods and how they are marketed.
- Learn what quality foods are and how to choose them.
- Find quality foods you *like*.
- Gradually replace processed foods and so-called diet foods with real foods you like.
- Long term: try to get to a point where 80 percent of your food intake is real food.

THE BATTLE OF QUANTITY

This is the final battle. It comes *after* the Battle of Quality because you can't easily regulate the quantity you eat if the quality of your food is poor. *Quality influences Quantity*!

Goals:
- Learn techniques to defeat outside influence (experts, friends, family, marketing, etc.) over how much you eat.
- Practice techniques to reawaken your internal appestat so you'll know when you are hungry and when you are full.
- Put your appestat in charge of how much you eat.

THE FINAL FRONTIER

The Final Frontier is not a battle: it's an epilogue. With the four battles completed you'll have a solid baseline: a body healed with quality foods and increased activity, tools to manage quantity, and a stable weight. That leaves only one goal:
- Apply a few simple techniques to help your body *gradually* lose weight and *keep it off.*

THE ORDER OF BATTLE

The order of the battles is important. You can't fight them all at the same time. Start with the Battle of the Mind. A few weeks into that, start the Battle of Activity. When you feel like you have a handle on the Battle of the Mind—when you have mostly defeated the diet mentality—start the Battle of Quality. *Do not* start the Battle of Quantity until you are at least 60 percent successful with the Battle of Quality. That's because quality foods satisfy and regulate your appetite and you can't hope to adjust your quantity without that internal satisfaction.

Everyone comes from a different dietary and activity background; you may find that some battles are harder or easier for you than others. Leverage your current strengths and concentrate your efforts on the battles you most need to win.

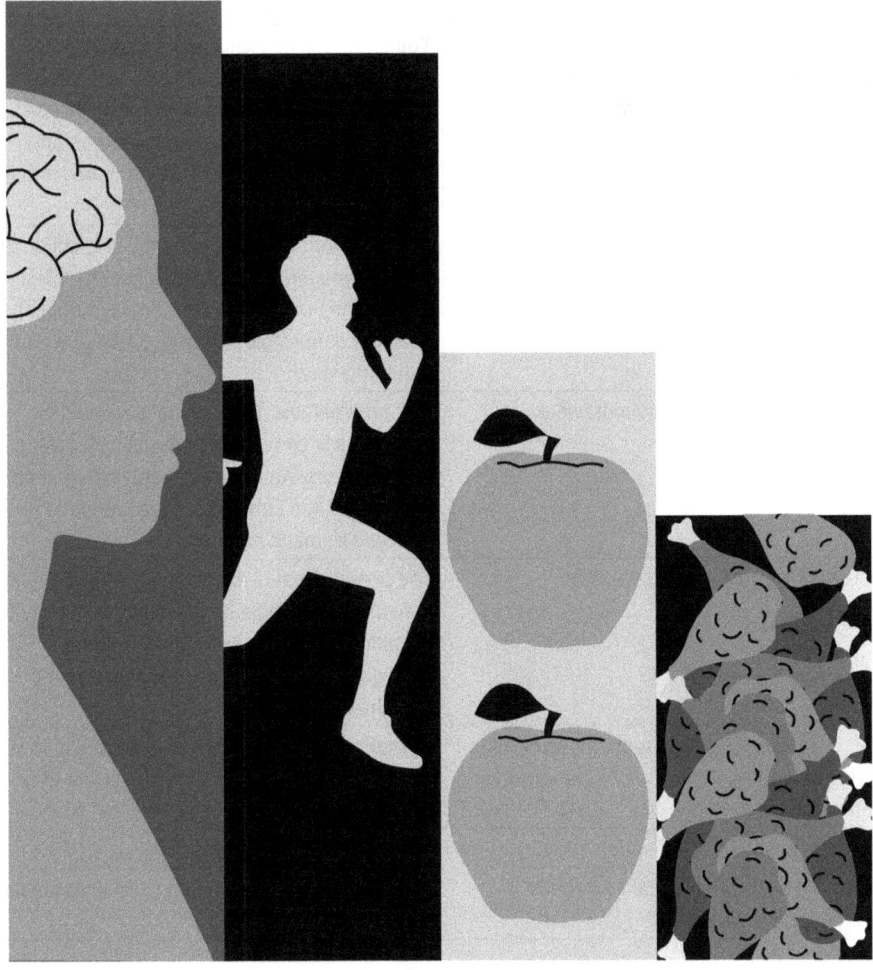

How is *Resetting Normal* different?

A COMPARISON

Here is a handy comparison where you can see the difference between *Resetting Normal* and ordinary diets.

Diet	Resetting Normal
Focuses primarily on measuring weight loss.	Does not measure weight loss.
Requires you to make major changes in your lifestyle in a short period of time.	You make only one or two changes at a time and do not move to the next until you're comfortable with the ones you've made. You set your own pace.
Sets unrealistic expectations for you.	Sets realistic, achievable expectations.
Requires you to modify both the quality and quantity of food at the same time.	You first adapt the quality of your food. Then you tackle the quantity problem.
Requires you to engage in an exercise program and tracks your progress by your weight loss and body measurements or BMI.	You engage in an exercise program in very small steps, getting comfortable with each step before you advance to the next. You do not track your weight or your measurements—exercise is not to lose weight but to become fit for life.
Requires you to immediately make major changes in what you eat.	You start with what you currently like, building on what you already eat that is healthy. Then you find healthy alternatives, one at a time, that you are comfortable with substituting for your unhealthy ones.
Has a timetable: lose x pounds/week.	Has no timetable. Progress is measured by looking back two or three months and asking the questions: Am I eating healthier now then I was then? Am I more fit? If the answer is yes, then you've made progress.
The primary goal is to lose weight.	The primary goal is to become healthier by permanently changing eating and activity behavior in such a way that it becomes the normal behavior. Weight loss can be a side effect of this change.
Requires unnatural food restrictions by specifying quantity, calories, fat, or carbohydrate intake.	Revitalizes your own internal appestat so that you can depend on your body to tell you what, how much, and when you need to eat.
Fosters feelings of deprivation.	Fosters feelings of satisfaction.
Does not deal with the real sources of hunger.	Attacks the sources of hunger at the metabolic level.

If you're still not convinced

Most diet plans will promise you that you can drop x pounds in the first two weeks and then x pounds/week thereafter. This kind of promise is not part of *Resetting Normal* because when you attack the real, underlying problem *the benefits accrue over time.* You may not see anything obvious for a while because the early changes are internal. Then, as you and your body adjust, the effect becomes visible—the change expands from the inside to the outside.

Here are just a few more reasons that make *Resetting Normal* worth the effort:

SMALL EFFORT PRODUCES HUGE PAYOFF

Resetting Normal is nearly effortless. You set small, achievable goals—not related to weight loss—which will get you where you need to go over time. This process works because as you make one change and get used to it, *your body changes in response.* Your tastes and your habits will evolve naturally if you don't force them. If you've ever wanted to be like one of those people who always seem to know when to stop eating and never think about dieting, you can be. I would never have believed I could be that way, but I am now, and it's one of the most satisfying and liberating feelings I know.

AN OUNCE OF PREVENTION—THE BEST INSURANCE YOU CAN BUY

Not everything can be fixed, which is why prevention is better. While physicians can do amazing things, *they can't fix everything.* Consider this Chinese proverb: *He who takes medicine and neglects diet wastes the physician's time.* Resetting Normal will show you that a lifestyle that fosters prevention doesn't have to be miserable. And at the end of *Resetting Normal* you'll find freedom and enjoyment, not continual denial.

While there are no guarantees that changing your lifestyle will keep you disease-free, doctors can't guarantee that their medical treatments will do that either. Consider what income you might have when you retire. Wouldn't you rather spend that on having a good time rather than on health care? What would it be like not to have to take pills every day, as many seniors do? Good food is far cheaper than medicine or health insurance, and physical activity can be totally free.

INSTANT GRATIFICATION DOESN'T LAST LONG

From personal experience I know that thinking long-term is difficult. All during my dieting phases I was so anxious to lose the weight I'd say to myself, "I'll just get this weight off and then I'll make some permanent changes." Well, the follow-up never happened because dieting never prepared me for long-term maintenance; I could never quite figure out how that worked. So in the words of LeBlanc's Law for software development, "Later equals never." We have good intentions, but somehow they get lost in the chaos of daily living. When I finally made that long-term commitment, it turned out to be the shortest path to the end goal.

YOU CAN DO THIS BEFORE IT'S MEDICALLY NECESSARY

It's amazing how a near-death experience can change a person's behavior for the better: someone has a minor heart attack and suddenly becomes interested in changing diet and exercise. But why wait? Sometimes there isn't a second chance. If you take care of it now, you can take your time. Rushing is your enemy because it takes time to make new habits become your normal. Small changes are easy to make permanent. Real, whole foods taste good and you won't feel deprived.

***RESETTING NORMAL* IS FLEXIBLE**

This approach does not espouse a specific diet other than gradually displacing processed foods with real, whole foods. What those whole foods are is entirely up to you and your taste preferences. When you become familiar with the wide array of great foods available to you, you might be amazed at your choices. You can be an omnivore, a vegetarian, or a vegan—whole foods work in any category.

Whatever your ultimate goal is, resetting your normal can help you.
- If your goal is to stop stressing about your diet and accomplish something productive in your life, this plan can take you there.
- If your goal is to lose weight, this plan can take you there.
- If your goal is to stop the cycle of gaining and losing weight, this plan can take you there.
- If your goal is to consume less fat, this plan can take you there.
- If your goal is to become a vegetarian or vegan, this plan can take you there.
- Whatever your goal, you can apply the process of *resetting normal* to help you.

If you have something that already works for you—if you're healthy and at a good weight and you're comfortable maintaining it—chances are you've *already reset your normal*; you just probably never thought of it that way. If not, and you're tired of diet games, maybe you're ready for a different approach. Quit banging your head against the wall—follow this transformation process now and be done with it. *Resetting normal* is a natural, permanent solution.

PART 3: THE PLAN
CHAPTER 7
THE BATTLE OF THE MIND

The Context

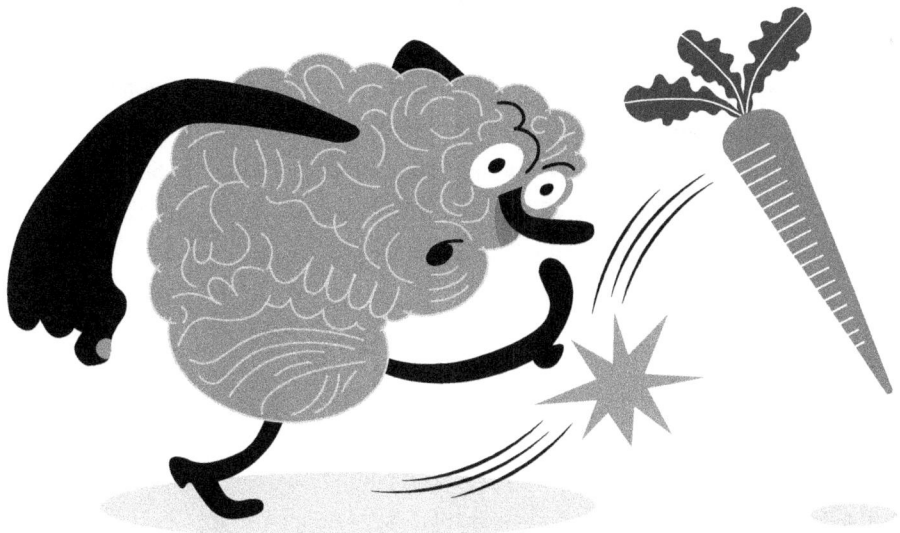

Even if you've never dieted, chances are you feel torn between what you think you *should* eat and what you *really* want to eat. And it's likely that you've become dependent on outside advice about what, when, and how to eat rather than paying attention to the signals your own body gives you.

You must to extricate yourself from this way of thinking to reset your normal. I had no idea how deeply embedded it was for me until I tried to escape. Through trial and error, I found some techniques that finally worked. I had to:

- Create the right environment
- Diet-proof myself
- Expert-proof myself
- Commercial-proof myself
- Social-proof myself

The purpose of this battle is to clear your brain of diet-centered thinking. With a clean slate you can tap into your own power over appetite regulation—your own internal appestat.

The Challenges

CREATE AN ENVIRONMENT FOR A NEW MINDSET

"Suspension of disbelief" is a concept typically applied to fiction, where the writer presents an implausible tale in such a way that the reader can temporarily believe it's true. Movies with superheroes come to mind as a good example. Suspension of disbelief can sometimes be a valuable tool in real life as well. If you're like I was, you don't believe you have any innate ability to guide your own eating habits. For you, the world of food is all about learning how to control yourself by applying the advice of someone else. I'm asking you, in the face of that belief, to believe the opposite—to believe you *do* have that natural ability. This process is equivalent to deprogramming the old way of thinking and learning to trust yourself—even if you need to pretend for a while.

Action #1: Put the scale out of reach

The first thing I'm going to ask you to do is take your scale and put it where you can't get to it easily. I didn't throw mine out, but I put in the deep dark recesses of the garage. Shocking? Not really, when you stop and think that people lived for millennia without measuring themselves this way. And here's why.

If you're a confirmed yo-yo dieter, here's a scenario you've probably been through many times:

Let's say you've been on a diet for three weeks and you feel REALLY good. More energetic, thinner. Absolutely great. And you can't wait for your weekly weigh-in—you're *sure* you've lost another two pounds. You can just feel it. You're excited about getting on the scale. Elated even.

Then you step on the scale ... Oops ... Wait ... This *can't* be right. It says you've actually gained a pound. You get off the scale and try again. Same result. You sigh, disappointed. You tell yourself it must be the exercise. You've been working out regularly and the experts say that muscle weighs more than fat, so you probably have more muscle now. Or maybe it's water weight. Yeah, that's got to be the reason. It has to be! You've been good and you've stuck to your diet absolutely.

You get off the scale. But now you don't feel so good. Not as energetic. And now that you think about it, you actually feel kind of fat. You should've known better than to imagine it was actually going to work this time. You tell yourself you'll keep at it, that it will correct itself by the end of the week. But no matter how you try to convince yourself of this you feel demoralized. You feel cheated. Betrayed. You've worked hard the last three weeks and all for nothing.

By the time you get to work you're in a really bad mood. You've tried to put a good spin on the situation but to no avail, and by mid-morning you're asking yourself, "What's the point?" You find an excuse to go for coffee and get tempted by some coffeecake. Might as well. Diet's not working anyway. Maybe you don't deserve to be thin. At least if you can't be thin you can be comforted eating something indulgent. Anyway, who cares?

What you don't realize is that by having unreasonable expectations and trying to measure yourself by them, you've set yourself up for a *superficial* failure. Ask yourself how you could possibly go from feeling great, energetic, and thin, to feeling awful, lethargic, and fat—all in the space of the few moments between pre-scale and post-scale. The truth lies with your pre-scale feeling. You *were* doing great, exactly on track, and the simple act of using the wrong measurement of success—weight—triggered you to sabotage yourself.

While experts are quick to point to studies showing that people lose more weight and maintain it better when they continually monitor themselves, that research assumes an environment of dieting and micromanagement. When you reset normal, you remodel your environment in such a way that you don't have to weigh yourself daily or watch every pound. Getting rid of the scale was the first thing I did, and I've never looked back. Despite that, I lost the weight I wanted to, and my weight has been stable for more than ten years. I only use my scale now to weigh my luggage before a flight.

If putting the scale out of reach makes you nervous, write down some of your worst fears in the online workbook for this Action. Then each week, note how your feelings change as you gain more confidence in living without this mechanical device to gauge your state of health.

Action #2: Hide the calorie charts and fat counting books

Diet experts have focused on weight-loss formulas that require keeping track of various food elements such as calories, carbohydrates, and fat so that you don't exceed some arbitrary daily maximum. Unfortunately, these formulas don't account for all the factors in real life that affect metabolism. More importantly, they don't consider that the *nutritional value of your food* is a much more important factor in controlling your consumption than adding up the calorie/fat/carb content and limiting yourself to arbitrary quotas.

The underlying belief on the part of diet experts is that we're all so broken, we can't possibly know what to eat or how much unless we micromanage. I bought into that belief myself all those years I was dieting. It didn't take long to realize I'd been counting calories, fat grams, and carbs for so long I knew them by memory. Removing the references was the easy part; ignoring the numbers stored in my head took a lot longer. Nevertheless, I made the effort to suppress that information whenever it popped into my mind, and over time I managed to stop thinking about food in terms of numbers.

So hide all those number-counting references. And that includes disabling the equivalent smart phone apps that tally calorie, fat, or carb totals daily. As you reset normal, you'll learn what and how much your body needs to be satisfied, and it will regulate itself. You'll have no need to calculate anything. The next time you want a particular food and you're tempted to look up how many calories or fat or carb grams it contains, DON'T.

DIET-PROOF YOURSELF

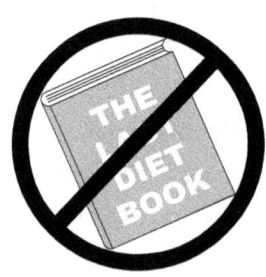

Despite more than one hundred years of various diet strategies, current obesity statistics clearly show that dieting is an ineffective method of losing weight. I've seen numbers ranging between 5 and 20 percent for dieters who maintain any weight loss—a dismal success rate. Not only do people fail to lose weight permanently, many of them actually gain weight, making the problem even worse, driving them into yo-yobesity. Logic should dictate that standard dieting advice is wrong because if the diet solution was correct, more people would succeed than fail.

Obesity is the result of being overfed and undernourished and behaving normally according to our Western lifestyle. Forcing someone to diet is an attempt to correct overfeeding by underfeeding without addressing the undernourished and cultural parts of the problem. Underfeeding won't fix anything because no one can tolerate it for very long.

Here are a few specific reasons why dieting fails:
- Dieting requires overriding your natural appetite through micromanagement.
- Dieting places artificial and unnatural limits on various food groups.
- Dieting fosters dysfunctional eating patterns.
- Dieting perpetuates the fallacy that thin = healthy.

- Dieting does not prepare you for maintenance.
- Dieting creates and perpetuates the denial-indulgence cycle that drives yo-yobesity.
- Diets focus on short-term results, not long-term results.

And here's one more that deserves a deeper explanation: dieting strategies are trendy and subject to change. When one theory doesn't seem to work, the experts trot out another one. As of this writing, the current focus is on calories. We are constantly told that if we burn more calories than we consume we'll lose weight—I call this "diet math." I also call it a fallacy because it doesn't always work that way. And here's why.

First, the definition of a calorie: a unit of energy-producing potential in food.

What is usually ignored is that this measure of energy has a different effect based on how it's *packaged* and how your body metabolizes it. A 200-calorie candy bar is processed differently in your body than 200 calories of carrots.

According to a law of physics, energy can the neither created nor destroyed. So theoretically, if you take in more calories than you burn, the potential energy from the excess calories has to get stored somewhere—as fat. And if you burn more calories than you take in, the energy for the burning has to come from somewhere (preferably some the stored fat). The diet experts tell us that there are 3,500 calories in one pound of fat. So if you burn 3,500 more calories than you need for maintenance, you should lose one pound. Now I'm not going to argue against this law of physics, but I am going to argue that the way it's applied to dieting is wrong because this is a *laboratory formula* based strictly on mathematics and not on your body's actual metabolism.

In reality, it's not that simple. If you follow this regimen, in one week's time, you might lose one pound and you might not. Or you might lose two. Or, quite possibly, you might gain one.

The reason? It's a short-term measurement. I don't care what the mathematicians or the physicists or the nutritionists say—you can't tell what your body is going to do *in the short term*. Your body processes different kinds of foods in different ways and at different rates. And your body has its own set of rules, foremost of which is maintaining what is called *homeostasis*—keeping itself in a stable, constant condition. When something happens that threatens that condition, it will move to compensate. For example, get too hot? Your body causes you to sweat, which then lowers your temperature. When you try to change things such as your weight, your body doesn't always cooperate. Some people can reduce calories to a very low level and ramp up exercise and still not lose weight. It's pretty easy to calculate calories consumed, but it's difficult to calculate calories expended. That's because there are other factors at work.

Metaphorically speaking, we all have a little metabolic gremlin, and it has a mind all its own. Cut your intake too drastically and it responds by *s-l-o-w-i-n-g* itself down and *r-a-m-p-i-n-g* your appetite up. It may become more and more efficient with the energy it expends. Let's say you eat 2,000 calories a day on average so when you go on a diet you cut that to 1,500. Your resident metabolic gremlin might just decide that if you're only going to give it 1,500, by George, it'll just figure out a way to get by on 1,500 instead of 2,000 without burning fat to make up for the missing 500. So you might not lose any weight even though it seems like you should. And then, to add insult to injury, when you abandon your diet and go back to your normal 2,000, you might actually gain weight because you'll be taking in 500 more calories than your gremlin now uses and it'll just stash those away as fat for future use.

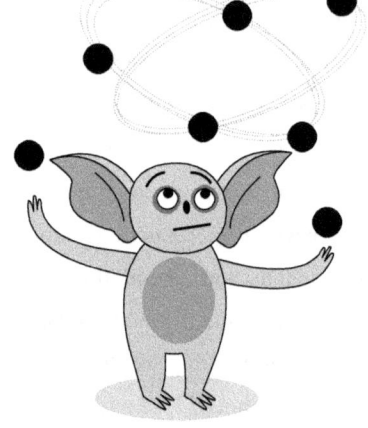

Need more evidence? Ever experience the weight plateau? Sometimes your metabolic gremlin just digs in and refuses to let you lose any weight at all. You may go on a diet and seem to be doing fine. Then you hit this virtual plateau where no matter how drastically you cut calories you can't drop any weight, until your body decides to let you. If losing weight were strictly a mathematical formula in action *minute by minute*, that wouldn't happen.

Now, to pacify the physicists and nutritionists out there, I can't argue with the fact that *over a long period of time*, if you *eat the right kinds of foods* and expend more calories than your body needs for maintenance you will lose weight. But how your body responds to calorie restriction from one week to the next is entirely unpredictable because you don't know day to day your body's caloric needs and what your metabolism is doing. Throw in some exercise that builds muscle, and that further complicates the process. The number of calories your body needs to burn just for maintenance is really a guesstimate; you have no way of knowing exactly what that number is, so you can't calculate with any certainty how many calories you need to cut out of your diet to lose a specific number of pounds in a week. It's impossible to predict exactly how your body will react in the short term.

I've lived through these scenarios many times over. And since scientists haven't yet figured out all the factors that allow your body to accomplish these dietary acrobatics, it seems obvious that reducing it to one simple formula is misleading and we shouldn't trust it.

Turning diet thinking on its head is not trivial. I had no idea how ingrained dieting was in my head until I tried to get it out. But I did succeed, and in this section I offer my strategies to help you do the same.

Don't blame yourself if you have failed in the past. Dieting is not a natural process. I learned from experience that dieting is not the solution to a weight problem—*it is part of the problem*. Consequently, one of the fundamental underpinnings of *Resetting Normal* is that *the practice of dieting has no place in healthy normal*

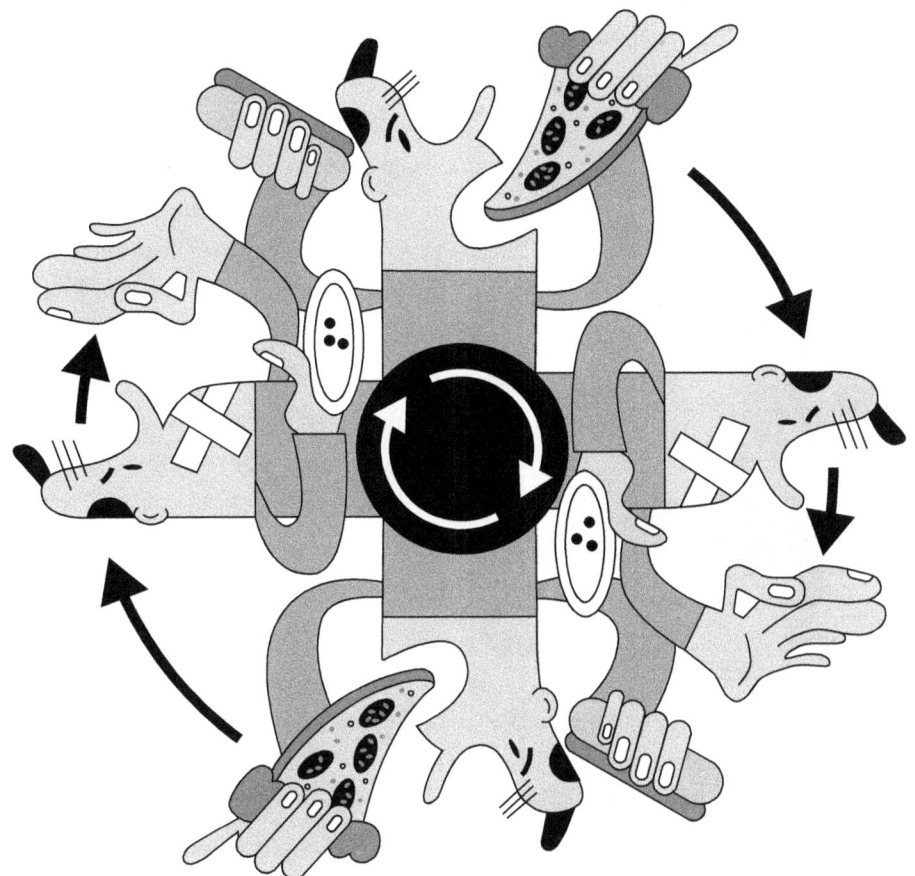

behavior. You simply must get rid of it. It drives yo-yobesity through the denial-indulgence cycle. *When you diet-proof yourself you avoid the dieting paradox:* dieting *promises* weight-loss but over the long term, *promotes* weight gain.

Once more, it leaves us feeling unsatisfied, guilty, and vulnerable to weight-loss scams. Here's how to exterminate this kind of thinking.

Action #3: Ditch the specific weight loss goals

In *Resetting Normal* you're not giving up setting goals, but your goals will be different—realistic and achievable. And when you're finished, you too will be like the tiny percentage of the population who knows intuitively how much to eat and when to stop, and who maintain an appropriate weight as easily as breathing.

Stopping dieting requires that you *ditch specific, time-driven* weight-loss goals. It's ok to keep in the back of your mind that your ultimate goal is to lose weight. But *do not get any more specific.* Committing yourself to lose twenty pounds in two months or five pounds in the first week puts you directly into diet mode. You'll start tracking what you eat and weighing yourself, and you'll be right back where you started—a short-term goal instead of a permanent solution.

The diet paradigm enforces mind over matter—you're supposed to use willpower to control your body and make it lose weight. The problem is that Body is not just a slave of Mind, Mind and Body are *partners*. You may be able to force Body to bend to your will in the short term but in the long term, Body will snap back and get even with you. To get the partnership going, you must stop trying to force your body to adhere to artificial time/weight-loss goals.

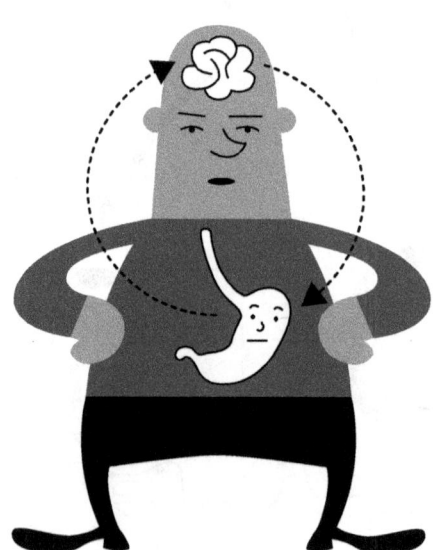

It may be hard at first not to use weight as a reference point. But if you just trust in the long term, you won't need this measurement, you'll actually begin to feel a huge sense of relief. The enormous diet gorilla that's been sitting on your shoulders all these years will just give up and go away. (Even if you haven't lost a single pound you'll feel a hundred pounds lighter.)

Remember that you're going to heal from the inside out. It's going to take some time to internalize a new relationship with food, but once you do, everything will fall into place. What you're going to do is gradually change what you like to eat and how much you eat. And the side effect of your success at this will be weight loss, if that is your intent.

Think of your Mind as the wise manager who listens to an employee and trusts that they are competent to do their job. Whenever you decide how much weight you will lose by [some specified time] you're being the mean, demanding boss, not the wise manager. To counter this kind of thinking, repeat the following every day:

"My Mind and Body are partners."

"If I listen, my body will tell me what it needs to be satisfied."

"If I listen, my body will tell me what it needs to lose weight."

Action #4: Give yourself permission to eat whatever you want

Yes, this is scary.

It is true that some foods are good for you (whole foods) and some are not (most processed foods). However, this phase of *Resetting Normal* is about conquering a dysfunctional psychological mindset, not about what you should or shouldn't eat. In the Battle of Quality, you'll engage in the process of replacing the bad stuff with healthy alternatives.

The primary reason this phase is scary is that based on your past eating experience—which probably has been defined by restrictive eating, guilt, and fear rather than normal eating—it's natural to fear that if you gave yourself the green light to eat ice cream (or chocolate chip cookies or bacon or whatever) anytime you wanted, you'd overdose on it. But …

Past and current experience will not necessarily determine future experience if your entire eating context is different.

By that I mean, once you move out of the I-can't-have-it stage into the I-can-have-it-anytime-I-want stage, you'll change your entire relationship with food.

But won't I be compromising my health by doing this? No, not in the long run. First of all, not everything on the standard forbidden-foods list is really bad for you when consumed in small quantities. There's a big difference between eating one piece of fried chicken and eating a bucketful, between eating one donut and eating three or four, between eating four ounces of steak and eating a one-pounder, between a couple of tablespoons of sour cream on your baked potato and a half a cup.

Also keep in mind that *this is only the first step in the process.* If you suffer from the denial-indulgence cycle, especially if you are prone to food binging, you need to go through this step to level out your eating behavior. You need to stop thinking of food in terms of punishment (denial) vs. reward (indulgence) because that's what drives the cycle. If you really want to get in control of what you eat, you need to take the forbidden attribute out of your food equation. Removing it will allow you to decide for yourself— based on your body's signals, likes and dislikes, food availability, and social situation—what, when, and how much you need to eat.

No doubt you have a long list of forbidden foods. Restrictive eating espouses too many don'ts: don't eat eggs, red meat, salt, saturated fat, cheese, fast food, donuts, dessert, salad dressing, ice cream, and so on. But removing all of them from your diet can set you up for both psychological and physical cravings. If you've grown up eating these things and you like them, giving them all up in one massive sweep is *way outside of your normal.*

The long-term goal is to find real, whole, satisfying and healthy foods that you'll come to like better than what you're eating now. But you can't reset normal successfully by trying to change them all at once. In the meantime, you set the stage for the resetting process with a little mental preparation: stop demonizing certain types of foods and give yourself permission to have what you like without guilt. The next step: some qualifying rules to minimize the impact.

The goal of this Action is to kick yourself out of the denial-indulgence cycle. When you deny yourself foods you really like you build up a craving for them, until one day it overflows and you eat yourself silly. This process can be a little tricky when you first start out because it's likely you're eating mostly processed foods, which fuel hunger in unnatural ways. But you can get through this safely with some precautions outlined in the next Action.

Action #5: Apply some limits

You can go through this process safely by applying some limits. Permission is *not* a license to eat two boxes of candy at a time or two pounds of steak or four Big Macs or whatever your food weakness happens to be. The way to do this is to set some limits for each encounter. Get it into your head that if you want more the next day you can have it. Instead of thinking, "This is bad for me; I shouldn't be eating it but as long as I am I might as well eat as much as I can now and then I'll make up for it by depriving myself for the next [three] months," think, "I can eat this anytime I want it so there is no need to pig out on it right now."

I understand that this idea runs counter to the usual advice, which dictates that if you want something experts say is bad for you, you should substitute something they say is better: if you crave ice cream, eat low-fat frozen yogurt instead; if you crave a cinnamon roll, look for one with reduced fat and artificial sweetener; if you are hungry for a snack, choose raw vegetables with low-fat dip; if you want toast with butter, get it with no butter or with low- or non-fat margarine. So why am I telling you it's ok to eat what you really want instead? Isn't that medically unsound?

No, and here's why.

First, this is a transition time, just the first battle—the Battle of the Mind.

Second, many of those substitutes are worse for you than the real thing because
- They are made from highly refined ingredients.
- They contain artificial ingredients and additives.
- They are less satisfying and not only are you likely to eat more, they won't stem your hunger for long.

Third, when you eat the real thing you want, when you want it:
- It's more satisfying and you can get by with less of it.
- You eat it and you're done with it, so you're not creating a dam of pent-up desire that will ultimately rupture and come crashing down on you.

The actual long-term goal is to reduce your consumption of highly processed foods. But you'll never meet that long-term goal unless you reduce your cravings for them. To reduce your cravings, you have to topple those foods off their throne of desirability. Put those foods in their place. Make them ordinary.

To get used to this kind of thinking, when you want something you *think* you shouldn't have, give yourself permission to eat it anyway—just stick to the standard serving size. And remind yourself you can have it tomorrow again, if you want—it's not a now-or-never decision. For example:
- Real bacon (not processed low fat turkey or beef bacon)—two pieces
- Whole eggs—two
- Real cheese (not low-fat, unless you happen to prefer it)—one to two ounces
- Beef—four to six ounces
- Donuts—one

Action #6: Defuse a binge

If you're the kind of person who tends toward binging on certain foods you crave, you can defuse this behavior by eating your binge food frequently in small amounts. This will put a cap on your cravings and the craziness that follows.

For example, let's say you love ice cream but refrain from eating it because you're on a diet. The pro-active anti-binge defense should depend on your reaction.

	Reaction	Anti-binge technique
Mild	You break down after a month and stuff yourself with a giant ice cream sundae as a reward for the month's denial.	Give yourself permission to eat one cup of your favorite ice cream once a week. Or a quarter cup four times a week.
Severe	You break down after only a week, or when some emotional event occurs, and you consume a half gallon of ice cream.	Give yourself permission to have a half cup of your favorite ice cream every day.

Yes, that's still a lot of ice cream in both cases, but the point is that when you get to eat this food often enough, it loses its specialness as a reward and there is no longer any point in binging on it. It's also likely that you'll just get tired of it after a while.

If you have a problem with binging, apply this technique to your problem binge food. Let yourself have some every day or every week—guilt-free.

Action #7: Prevent a binge

It's possible to prevent binges altogether rather than trying to defuse them. It's the same concept—allowing yourself to eat what you like—but in this case you put a beautiful fence around your consumption by creating a ritual where you can relax and enjoy your food regularly, guilt-free.

To do this, choose a regular time and place to enjoy your special food—Friday night pizza, Sunday morning pancakes once a month, mocha latte on a Saturday afternoon—whatever it is, decide on a reasonable quantity, eat and enjoy it, and then look forward to the next scheduled event.

Action #8: Minimize the effect of sugary foods

Foods high in sugar are particularly tricky to deal with. That's because sugar triggers a strong insulin response that can make you even hungrier than you were before you ate it. How can you feel comfortable giving yourself permission to eat sweet foods whenever you want? One way is that you don't eat them first or by themselves. Eat something else first and then go ahead, guilt-free, within limits. Think dessert: there's a reason it's small and comes at the end of dinner rather than the beginning.

If you usually start your day with a soda or a donut—don't. You can still have it, but have some eggs, cheese, bacon, toast with cream cheese, or even lunch meat first. If you usually have cookies or candy for a snack in the afternoon or late evening, try eating cheese or fruit (apple, grapes, pear, etc.) first. Then, eat your sweet if you still want it, but eat less of it. This Action is just the first step in reducing your overall sugar consumption.

Action #9: Start communicating with your body

Once you are comfortable with your food limits and have binging under control, it's time to begin to reawaken your own internal appestat. You do this by establishing communication with your body. Instead of telling it what/when/how much to eat, ask it.

When you get hungry, ask yourself what you *really* want. At that moment of hunger, if you didn't have your brain loaded with rules about what you're supposed to eat and what you're supposed to avoid, if you could choose anything in the world to eat, what would it be? Then ask yourself: Is it protein? Is it fatty? Is it sweet? Is it salty? Is it a vegetable? Is it [whatever]? Obviously, you'll have to narrow it down to what's available to you at the time, but it's likely that even if the specific item you want isn't available, there will be something available in the same category. Once you figure out what that is, then eat it. And don't feel guilty about it. Just don't eat a ton of it. Remind yourself that you can eat more of it later if you want to—later that day or tomorrow or whenever—so you don't have to eat it all *now*.

At first you may have some difficulty zeroing in on just what it is that your body is asking for. But it's a learning process, and you'll get better at it pretty quickly. Even if you can't get that particular food at that moment, it's instructive to try to interpret your body's feedback.

Action #10: Give yourself permission to eat when you're hungry

Experts have doled out conflicting rules regarding when and how often you should eat. Here are a few of the most common ones:

- Always eat breakfast.
- Instead of three meals per day, graze on six or more small snacks throughout the day.
- Eat something before you exercise.
- Don't eat at night.
- Don't skip meals.

I can replace all those with just one rule:

- Eat only when you're hungry.

The reason the experts' formulas are misleading is that they can't take into consideration the state of your mind or your metabolism at any given moment. Only *you* can know when you're hungry and when you're full. And that isn't necessarily going to be at the same time every day. Your hunger might be on one schedule during the workweek and a different one on the weekend, and it will vary based on your stage of life. If you are a single adult workaholic, your hunger schedule will be different from that of a working mother, and different still if you are a senior citizen. Or you might just decide one day that you want to try something different.

Here's my personal reaction to the experts' rules above:

The edict to eat breakfast: Usually I do, but if I've had a large meal the night before (maybe dinner out), I might not be hungry in the morning so I might skip it altogether, or I might wait and have a small mid-morning snack. If I'm not hungry in the morning, I don't eat.

The edict to graze: I'm not a fan of the grazing style of eating. That's because with that method I'm never full long enough to stop thinking about food. Is it time for my next snack? Is it time for lunch? I try to eat enough at each meal so that I'm comfortably full for the next three or four hours. That way I can focus on other things I want to do and forget about eating. Then, after three or four hours, my stomach gently reminds me it's getting hungry again.

Besides, finding healthy foods for the main three meals is hard enough. Carting around enough healthy food for frequent grazing would mean major planning ahead. How many snacks will I need? Will I be in a meeting when I get hungry? Will there be refrigeration so I could pack some protein? If not, what can I safely take? Am I taking the bus to work and if so, can I lug a cooler of food along with everything else I need to take? What about food bars? If you can find ones that have only fruit and nuts with no added sugar, other additives, or genetically modified ingredients, ok. Otherwise, sorry, they're not real food. They're simply candy bars given a healthy aura via a marketing campaign. In short, eating frequently complicates eating healthy food. That said, this is just how I feel about it. If the grazing style suits you, by all means do it.

The edict to eat before exercise: I generally don't, but that's because I usually exercise early in the morning. I have learned through experience that if I'm going to eat before exercise, it has to be at least a half hour or more before, and because I'm reluctant to get up early enough to do that, I just get by on whatever my body's got left over from the night before. Is this optimal? I don't know, but it seems to work for me. If it fits your schedule to eat before, it's probably a good idea. If not, don't worry about it.

The edict to not eat at night: I don't, but that's because I'm a morning person and I don't usually stay up late. Lots of people are just the opposite. My take is that as long as you only eat when you're genuinely hungry, there's nothing wrong with it. However, a number of other considerations might influence your decision on this. Are you just mindlessly eating because you've been prodded by commercials? Are you prone to acid-reflux problems? Do you have problems falling asleep? If the answer to any of those questions is yes, then you should try to eat dinner early and consume just enough that you're not hungry later.

The edict to not skip meals: Generally I don't, but the guiding principle is still *only eat when you are hungry.* You'll probably find that your eating times follow certain patterns and you'll have your best success at keeping satisfied if you stick with those patterns. However, there is one mitigating factor we can't avoid in our modern life: hectic schedules. If you're going to skip a meal, make sure you can last all the way through until the next one, or take some satisfying snacks. Otherwise, you'll be running on empty and heading for the vending machine.

If everything goes normally ... you're home free—just follow your normal eating pattern.

The gist of this Action is to put external rules aside and start listening to your body so you can apply the only rule that matters: *only eat when you're hungry.* It may be hard to tell at first whether you're truly hungry or you're just feeling some unnatural craving. But it's important in the process to ask the question and give it your best try at an answer.

Action #11: Continue communicating with your body

This adds another dimension to Action #10: When you're tempted to eat, ask yourself if you're *really* hungry or just responding to outside cues. (Is it time for lunch? Someone announces, "Donuts in office #5!" You've been told you should never skip breakfast. Food commercials ...)

Get into the habit of asking yourself the question: "Am I really hungry right now?" You might not be able to tell at first, and you might have trouble resisting the social implications of not eating when everyone else is, but at least pose the question, "Will I feel better or worse if I eat this now?" Try to focus on your internal fullness meter, then take a stab at an answer.

Action #12: Anticipate a food drought

If you anticipate a food drought sometime during the day ... Make sure you eat enough satisfying food when you can. If I know there will be a significant part of my day where I either won't have access to food at all or I will only have access to junk food, I'm going to eat enough of a meal beforehand that I won't be hungry. For example, when I travel a long distance (by car or plane) I will start the day with a large breakfast that includes highly satisfying foods like eggs, bacon, bread with butter, fruit, and a latte. After that, I'm good for anywhere up to six or seven hours without anything else. Same thing if I'm going to be stuck in a long meeting, a class, or an all-day conference. It beats having to carry around a gazillion snacks, and I don't ever have to worry about being stuck starving with nothing substantial to eat.

When it seems like the universe is out to get you ... To mitigate problem days when your schedule is sabotaged by unexpected events (extra late meeting at work, medical emergency for a family member, squirrels got into your house and tore up your furniture ...) and you can't maintain your normal eating routine, it's best to have some backup ammunition. By that, I mean have some substantial snacks handy. In the Battle of the Mind, you shouldn't be too concerned yet with what's on the good list and what's on the bad list, but some snacks will fill you up better and longer than others and need little or no refrigeration. Anything with a high fat content will last you longest. Consider peanut butter, apples, single-serving cheese slices, nuts, or hard-boiled eggs (in the shell). Don't worry too much about *what* at this point—just make sure you have something that you like will keep you going, even if it's a chocolate-nut bar.

This is important because before you have completely reset normal, it's likely that you'll still be consuming too much processed food that won't sustain you over long hours or under stress. You need to be fortified so that you don't have a precipitous drop in blood sugar or feel driven to head for the nearest vending machine. After you've reset normal and your body has had time to heal and stabilize, you'll be able to tolerate long periods without food. I am continually surprised at how little I need to eat to sustain myself for hours. But it took time for my body to get to that point.

You can only find out the right schedule for yourself through experimentation. When you start listening to your body's signals instead of someone else's rules, you'll quickly learn when you need to eat and when you do not. The problem is that you're just out of practice at doing that. Your hunger regulator (appestat) has been deactivated from misuse and abuse. Give it a chance and it will wake up again.

Action #13: *Fight the clear-the-deck mentality*

As yo-yo dieters, we've all done it. For years, every time we decided to start a diet on Monday that meant a farewell-food party the weekend before. If we weren't going to allow ourselves to eat donuts for the next four months we figured we deserved a final fling. And we had to get rid of any potential temptations. Now that you have the tools to allow yourself to eat whatever you want, whenever you want, there is no need for this behavior. There should be no, "I'm going on a diet on Monday." But how do you purge this thinking from your mind? If you're like me you've done this so many times it's just a natural reaction. Here's how I put a stop to it.

First, I left whatever temptations I had in the house, in place. Then, if there was something left over at the end of the weekend, such as cookies, I didn't let myself finish them off on Sunday night. Instead, I told myself that I could eat one or two on Monday, one or two on Tuesday, one or two every day until they were gone. And I made myself follow

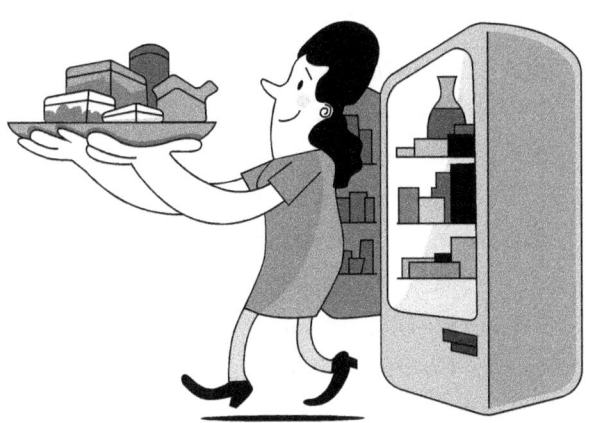

through on that. It felt wrong and I felt guilty. But I did it. Same process for any other formerly forbidden food, like pie or ice cream or potato chips—a small serving every day if I wanted, until it was all gone, or I got tired of it.

I understand if your initial reaction to this is that it seems very unhealthy. If nothing changed about my eating habits over many months, I would agree. But by making myself do this, within two months I eliminated my weekend-overindulgence, weekday-starvation cycle. And what happened more and more frequently was that I got tired of the goody before I'd eaten it all. As a result, I didn't consume as much of that formerly forbidden food and my overall consumption leveled out. Pre-diet binging became a thing of the past.

The reason it's so important to get rid of this mentality is that if you're yo-yo dieting, chances are that when you go through this clear-the-deck indulgence followed by dieting denial multiple times, what you consume with the indulgence overpowers what you give up with the denial, and you just gradually keep gaining weight. You are caught in the yo-yobesity trap.

To purge this behavior when you've been doing it for years, you need to force yourself to respond in a different way. Do the following at the end of every weekend and holiday:

- Do *not* get rid of diet-forbidden goodies in your house by eating them all at once or throwing them out.
- Decide on a reasonable portion size for them and dole them out to yourself a little every day until they're gone or you're tired of them.
- Resist feeling guilty.

Repeat this Action at the end of every weekend and every holiday. It will take time, but eventually you'll let go of your clear-the-deck mentality.

Action #14: Stop using food as a reward

Try to get yourself out of the habit of using special treats as rewards for denial. You should never say, "I've been good today, so I deserve a [sundae, donut, cheesecake, Venti Triple Caramel Macchiato with whipped cream and extra caramel ...]." It may not seem like it, but there is a difference between, "I got a raise today so let's go out for a nice dinner," and "I lost ten pounds so let's go out for a nice dinner." The first implies a celebration—which is ok. The second implies a justification to indulge after a denial and indicates a longing to go back to what used to be normal.

Food is food—that's it. There are times where food can be special, as for holidays, birthdays, and other celebrations. And that's ok. Some foods are associated with those days and they give more pleasure because of that: certain kinds of cookies for Christmas, potato pancakes for Hanukkah, cake for a birthday, a big dinner out for a celebration. But they are special because you only have them on those occasions. They do not serve as a *food reward*.

There might be a food you're particularly fond of that you think is forbidden. Let's say, for example, you like mac and cheese. Don't refrain from eating it (trying to be good) and then reward yourself with it when you feel like you have been good long enough. Make a ritual of having a reasonable serving of it once a week as a side dish. Look forward to it and enjoy it: "It's Thursday—my day for mac and cheese!" Don't look at it as a reward for not eating it the rest of the week; just enjoy the moment without guilt.

This is a subtle psychological action but an important one. When you allow yourself to eat what you want, when you want it, food loses its reward/punishment attribute, allowing you to regain control of your eating overall.

Action #15: Stop making yourself miserable

Food should not make us feel miserable. Healthy food does not have to be limited to oatmeal and egg whites or skinless, boneless chicken breast flavored only with herbs and lemon juice, or nonfat artificially sweetened yogurt. There are plenty of other options that are both healthy and tasty. When you feel you can enjoy the foods you like, even if in small quantities, you can regain some of the pleasure associated with eating. And you'll stop making yourself feel miserable. You'll become more satisfied with what you're eating and less likely to get depressed and go into an eating binge.

For this Action, make a list of all the foods that would make you happier if you could eat the real thing and then when you're hungry, choose foods you enjoy even if you've been brainwashed to think they're not healthy. Eat a small quantity and push back on the guilt. It's a mental process, but it will get easier.

There are many foods I still love to eat, including bread and butter, mashed potatoes, apple pie, chocolate, and others. However, I no longer *crave* them, nor am I tempted to binge on them. I enjoy them all the more because I don't eat them all the time. So don't think that after you reset normal you can never eat the foods you love. *Loving a food is not synonymous with craving it.* And you don't have to be miserable to be healthy.

EXPERT-PROOF YOURSELF

Action # 16: Block expert diet advice for a while

Experts have been telling us what to eat and how much for decades. But as more information is discovered, their advice changes. Study results have a way of being reversed years later (Coffee bad! Coffee good!). And what starts out as the result of one scientific study—useful to scientists as a piece of the puzzle in the whole metabolic process—gets transformed into an unproven health edict marketed to the public as a must-do.

For example, in the 1980s and 1990s, experts so demonized fat that many people came to think it should be avoided at all cost—even the fat in nuts, avocados, and fish. I was in a fish store once when two women came in looking for low-fat fish. The fishmonger, whose display case was filled with beautiful fresh salmon and halibut, tried to explain to them that the fat in fish is healthy, but they didn't believe him and left without buying anything.

This doesn't mean *all* expert advice is bad, but considering experts have since reversed their position on these types of fats, the switch should make you wonder what else they got wrong. To be successful in resetting your normal, you need to become your *own* expert—and you can by learning to listen to your own internal signals. The first step in accomplishing that goal is turning off the external advice.

Avoiding the continuous flow of external food directives is like trying to run between raindrops, but it is *possible*: you simply stop reading and listening. Temporarily:

- Put away the magazines and books that tell you what, when, and how much to eat.
- Stop listening to media reports that tell you what, when, and how much to eat (there's always the mute button).
- Stop visiting internet sites that tell you what, when, and how much to eat.

Action #17: Question conventional wisdom

Conventional wisdom is a generally accepted theory or belief. But generally accepted does not necessarily mean true. Today our health-related conventional wisdom travels the following path: results of scientific studies ➔ affirmation by public and private health organizations (experts) ➔ repetition through media exposure.

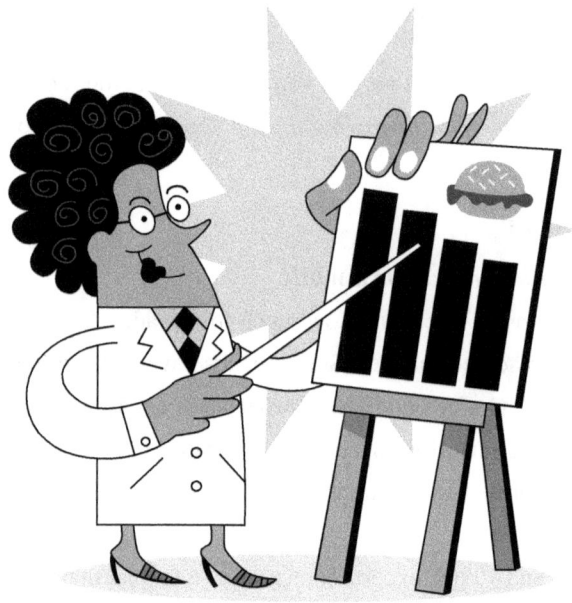

Driven by this process, our conventional wisdom includes rules that are incorrect. Worse, the biggest danger of conventional wisdom is that once you decide something is true, you close your mind to other possibilities whether or not the one you've latched onto is valid. Here are a couple of examples and why they are false.

"You can't be overweight and still be healthy." NO. First of all, this assumption depends on the definition of overweight. Experts have restricted the healthy weight range so that they can convince us that over a third of the population is obese [10]. If someone is *extremely* overweight he/she is very likely at risk for degenerative diseases. But as you get closer to the middle of that range, the benefits of losing weight

become a lot less significant. In fact, there has been more than one study showing that as we get older, a few extra pounds can actually be a benefit. So trying to lose that last ten pounds to meet experts' statistical requirement can be counter productive.

This factoid is another attempt to reinforce the false idea that thin = healthy. It also ignores two other important aspects of health: which foods make up a person's diet, and how fit that person is. If someone is thin because of an eating disorder, he/she is not healthy. If someone is thin but eats mostly junk food, he/she is not healthy. On the other hand, if someone ten or even twenty pounds over the medically approved limit eats a lot of vegetables and fruits and a reasonable amount of animal protein, limits sugar and refined carbs, includes healthy fats like olive oil and nuts, and is physically active, that person can be quite healthy[11].

"Fat-free food = fat-free body." NO. This is a myth. The supposed benefits of fat-free products win top honors in the flawed-conventional-wisdom sphere. At some point an expert coined the phrase "Only fat can make you fat," and thereafter fat-free products became everyone's salvation. There's just one little problem the experts didn't tell us: your body can only use a limited amount of carbohydrates, and when you exceed that, your metabolism starts storing them as saturated fat[12]. Since all those fat-free products are loaded with extra carbs—extra sugar in particular—if you're avoiding fat by substituting fat-free foods you're likely overloading your system with the kind of carbs your body will turn into the very thing you're trying to avoid[13].

This Action is a thought process. Whenever you hear some factoid over and over, ask yourself, "How do we know that's really true?" or "How did we come to blindly accept that information?" Try to think of exceptions you've observed personally. Scientists call these personal exceptions anecdotal evidence and they don't carry the weight of a full study, but it's still valid to bring them up.

Action #18 (optional): Find evidence that refutes conventional wisdom

There are plenty of other bits of questionable conventional wisdom floating around. Instead of assuming they're true, do a little research to find contrary evidence. You might consider scrutinizing any of the following, or find your own.

- The only way to lose weight is to limit calorie intake.
- The best eating pattern is vegetarian.
- Red meat is bad for you.

- Turkey bacon is healthier than regular bacon.
- Running is great for your health.
- Soy is the healthiest protein source.

If you decide to take this action, here are a few books that will help you. More are listed in the Resources section.

- *Fat Politics*, J. Eric Oliver
- *Health at Every Size*, Linda Bacon
- *The Whole Soy Story*, Kaayla T. Daniel
- *Wrong: Why experts keep failing us*, David H. Freedman

Action #19: Build confidence in yourself

It's ok to be a little defensive about the experts' dietary advice. I am by nature a non-confrontational, easy-going person. But after forty-three years of trying one dietary expert's plan after another, in good faith—putting significant effort into each one, I might add—and continually failing, I realized it was all for nothing. Nothing! Zip, zero, nada! Every single time I ended up right back at square one—my fat square.

I think you and I have every right to be skeptical. No one completely understands the big picture of food/weight/metabolism interaction yet, but that doesn't stop anyone from giving us directions according to what they think, based on the latest trendy study. There seems to be little recognition of individual differences or the sophisticated biological machinery the body uses to manage itself. We are *not* standardized products that roll off an assembly line. We come in an infinite variety of biological forms and our requirements are *not* all the same.

I would say to them, "Who are you to tell me what, when, and how much to eat? You're not inside my body monitoring my metabolism. You don't know what's going on in there. You can understand in general how cell metabolism works, but you cannot see exactly what is happening inside *me* when I eat or exercise or get hungry or stressed or tired. Even *I* can't determine *exactly* what's going on. But I *can* learn to read the signals and make helpful adjustments. *You can't* because you are on the outside. So there!"

What good does this skepticism do? It helps you have confidence in yourself. It helps you stop being a victim of dieting scams. It helps you to stop blaming yourself for failing to achieve *goals someone else has set for you using a method that has been proven over and over to fail*. It helps you to say No! to the diet mentality.

COMMERCIAL-PROOF YOURSELF

I'll say the same thing about product marketing claims that I have about experts' advice: if you want to be successful in *resetting normal*, you must to learn to listen to your body's own signals. The onslaught of product marketing claims that comes to us from all directions 24/7 has contributed to the evisceration of our respective appestats.

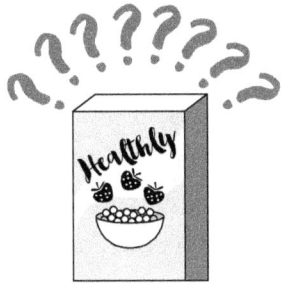

Most of us believe that we don't pay any attention to commercials or advertising. However, *a considerable number of us must be paying attention* or the food industry would not pour billions of dollars into advertising. In her book, *Food Politics*[14], academic nutritionist Marion Nestle describes what happened in 1984 when Kellogg displayed on its All-Bran cereal box a recommendation from the National Cancer Institute to "eat high-fiber foods." The implication was that eating All-Bran would help prevent cancer. Wrote Nestle, " ... [when] an FDA analysis revealed an astonishing 47 percent increase in the market share of All-Bran within the first six months of the campaign, the message to the food industry was clear: Health claims sold products."

Fight such psychological manipulation with the following actions.

Action #20: Become a skeptic—reject advertising claims

Start with the assumption that product-marketing claims are *almost always misleading.* The manufacturer wants you to buy their product and will try their best to put a healthy spin on it whether it's good for you or not. That does *not* make manufacturers evil, but *it does put the onus on us* to verify or debunk their claims. I'm *not* against advertising. I like to know what products are out there, what's new, and what's been changed. But I refuse to be lulled into passive acceptance of a product based on the manufacturer linking it to something supposedly healthy.

This action is a simple mental exercise: when you are confronted with a marketing claim, asked yourself the following:
- Does the claim seem reasonable?
- The manufacturer's goal is to make as much as money as possible from selling the product. But what's in it for you?
- Is the product a truly healthy alternative, or is the manufacturer using so-called health words to draw your attention away from other unhealthy aspects of it?

Action #21: Become a food-value label reader

The Battle of Quality takes up the labeling issue in detail. For now, just start getting in the habit of critically evaluating the packaging as it's presented. The list of ingredients is more important than the fat and calorie counts. I realize this can be a time-consuming activity, so tackle it a little at a time. Start with the items you use the most. Each time you go to the supermarket, pick one or two and consider the following guidelines:

- Don't look only at the calorie and fat counts—food has much more nutritional value than those statistics tell you.
- Don't get distracted by the health claim on the front of the package. A package may boast that it's organic on the front, while the list of ingredients on the back reveals it contains a high sugar and salt content. The quality of being organic will not make up for that.
- Do look at the ingredient list to see what artificial elements it contains. If the list is long, think twice about buying it. See the *Appendix C: Additives and Preservatives*.
- Try to figure out *what they don't tell* you about the product. A bread described as multi-grain gives the impression that it's a whole-grain product. But ingredients are listed in order of proportion by weight, so if the first ingredient is enriched bleached flour, it isn't very "whole."

I know how hard it is to separate fact from fiction in today's environment. We want to eat the right things to keep ourselves and our families healthy, and that makes us vulnerable to manufacturers' health claims. But reading the labels is a good start on an effective defense.

SOCIAL-PROOF YOURSELF

My 80/20 principle (if 80 percent of the food you eat is whole, the other 20 percent won't kill you) is designed to ward off fanaticism on your part. If you eat with others occasionally, it isn't going to hurt you to eat what they provide. There might be a few items you just don't want to eat anymore, but in my experience there's usually enough variety that avoiding one or two of them will go unnoticed. For example, I don't make a big deal out of it, but I don't drink soda—it tastes terrible to me now—but I'd also never announce, "I hate soda. I don't understand how anyone can drink that stuff." If there's no alternative like wine or beer, I might say I'm really thirsty and I'd just like to have some water.

Social pressure can take many forms. People tend to want you to eat and enjoy the same things they do. They also like you to validate their choices; if they feel like splurging with an ice cream sundae, they feel better if you join them. In general, they assume that others are aligned with the standard Western lifestyle. If you start to do something different, you may encounter disapproving reactions. They might be subtle, or they might be mean. If someone doesn't think you're eating according to whatever doctrine they think is correct, they may well put you down—maybe not to your face, but to others. Or they'll do it online for all the world to witness.

Action #22: Remain steadfast but low-key

It's all well and good for you to gradually switch from mostly processed foods to mostly real, whole foods. But that doesn't mean the rest of your social circle is doing the same thing—which puts you at odds with everyone else's normal. You'll still have to deal with the standard processed foods served by relatives, friends, the workplace, picnics, conferences, potlucks, and every other venue you can think of. Most of them mean well, so I've found that the best way to handle this situation is to stay low-key. If you get an invitation and you respond with a list of your new food preferences, you'll put an extra burden on your host.

If you like what they're serving and it falls in your 20 percent, eat it, enjoy it, and don't worry about it. If it's spills over into your 80 percent, *contribute something* if possible; bring a dish to share that fits your new food tastes. You can deliver it with a smile: "I thought you might enjoy this—it's a new recipe I've tried," or "I wanted to contribute something to the occasion." This way you'll have something you feel comfortable eating, and you can have small amounts of whatever your host provides without making a big deal out of it. And who knows—your host or other guests may love it. As long as this situation doesn't occur so frequently that it will sabotage you altogether, don't worry about it.

Action #23: Avoid a health-nut aura

If you waltz into someone's house for dinner and announce, "I don't eat that anymore" or deliver a lecture on the evils of processed foods, you not only insult your host, you set yourself up as a health nut. Which will make it harder for you because it's likely they'll target you as someone to reform—to bring you back to *their normal*. Instead of being direct and demanding, you can use more subtle ways to adapt.

Staying low-key, as in Action #22, will help. But there's still a chance that after a while you'll get labeled as a health nut anyway, because some people will start to notice that you don't eat the same way they do. If you eat small quantities of butter, steak, real mac and cheese, and so on—foods generally not considered healthy—and refuse desserts, donuts and cookies, or they catch you reading a label, sooner or later, someone will take notice.

The best response remains: don't make waves. Be as vague as you can about why you're making different choices. Some potential responses:

"I just feel like having this [whatever] today."

"I'm just curious about what's on the label."

"Dinner was fantastic! I think I'm too full for dessert right now."

Action #24: Blend in with social attitudes

Deviating from the norm is never easy. But you don't have to give up your friends to reset your normal. There are a couple of approaches you can take. I suggest you respond in one of the following ways:

Be quiet. You don't have to outwardly disagree with your social circle while you are make your own changes. You can temporarily pretend everything's the same. If they're discussing the latest diet fad, you don't have to contribute anything substantive. Just nod here and there and make non-committal noises like you would if you were on the phone with someone who keeps talking and talking and never gives you a chance to respond. But do listen because it's always good to know what other people are thinking, even if you don't agree.

Be mysterious. If your social circle tries to pressure you into doing what they're doing, just tell them politely that you're trying something different and you'll let them know later how it turns out.

Handling social media. If you're criticized on social media, take comfort in the fact that sooner or later, everyone is. It's something we'll all have to live with now and in the future. The best thing to do is to ignore it or drop off for a while. Don't let the sociopathic trolls control you.

Assume a quiet confidence. Just as with expert-proofing yourself, to reset normal you must to block out the external signals that override your internal ones. That includes what your family and friends say. Act like you know what you're doing and try not to be confrontational.

Measuring Success

The Battle of the Mind will be an ongoing project. You can defeat the diet mentality and forget about it, but you'll never be able to erase all the expert, social, and commercial pressures. They will continually evolve in their quest to control you, and you'll have to adapt your methods to counter them. It isn't necessary to completely win this war before moving on to the next phase. But you should at least get through the diet-proof stage. Don't worry if you still have some cravings and small binges. When you are eating mostly processed foods, your body doesn't have what it needs and it's going to complain about it in ways that don't make sense. The upcoming Battle of Quality will get you over that problem.

How long it takes you to diet-proof yourself will depend on the depth of your indoctrination in the diet mentality. It took me about 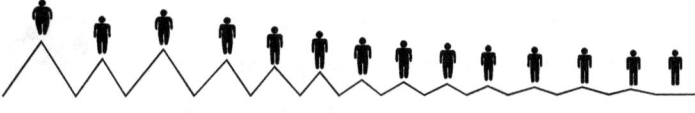 two months. Your transformation may take less time or more. But this is a hugely important step. If you are a confirmed yo-yo dieter, when you get to the point where you have put a stop to your denial-indulgence cycle, your eating patterns are mostly level, and you're not feeling guilty about everything you put into your mouth, celebrate your success. You are on your way *to resetting normal.* You are on your way to defeating yo-yobesity!

NOTES

CHAPTER 8
THE BATTLE OF ACTIVITY

The Context

WHY PHYSICAL ACTIVITY IS IMPORTANT

Ask yourself, "What are your personal goals?"

Do you want to be a doctor, a writer, a great parent, an artist, a musician, the best plumber ever, or a community volunteer? Whatever it is, putting exercise in perspective will allow you to be reasonably physically fit while freeing you up to meet your main life goals. Note that I am specifically *not* making any mention of losing weight as a goal of physical activity or formal exercise.

Here are the four principles I espouse in that regard:

- Physical activity is strictly for getting and keeping fit—physically and mentally.
- You may or may not lose weight as a side effect, but you should never judge the effectiveness of your activity routine by how much weight you have or have not lost.
- **Don't** exercise to lose weight.
- **Do** exercise to keep your infrastructure sound and gain all the benefits that exercise engenders.

THE SCIENTIFIC EVIDENCE

You don't have to look far to find numerous studies showing the benefits of exercise. Most of the experts who try to motivate people to engage in an exercise program cite these studies and explain the benefits of exercise on the circulation system, the heart, weight, hormones, the brain, and many other parts of the body. I haven't encountered *any* studies that show that *moderate* exercise is harmful in any way. Even if you are severely limited because of illness or disability, some type of body movement can be beneficial. If you think about it, the benefits of physical movement are self-evident.

HIGHLIGHTING THE OBVIOUS

Just take a moment to think about all living creatures. One thing they all have in common is that they *move* in some way. Even a simple amoeba moves, and even creatures attached to rocks use some movement to capture and eat their food. They *have* to move to live. Consequently, as little as they might move, if for some weird reason they stopped moving—just suppose they decided they didn't want to—they would deteriorate and die.

Now think about higher level animals. Monkeys swinging from trees. Mountain goats taking seemingly impossible leaps on the sides of cliffs. Squirrels in constant motion, scampering up and down trees and through the branches. Cheetahs that can run as fast as cars. Dolphins swimming in the ocean currents, leaping out of the water to great heights. How can you not be amazed by their physical abilities? Yet if for some weird reason, they stopped moving—again, just suppose they decided they didn't want to—they would deteriorate and die.

Now think about us human beings. Our brains and bodies are capable of an amazing variety of movements and physical feats. Olympic athletes, professional dancers, marathon runners, circus performers defying gravity with grace and balance, musicians whose fingers dart over strings and keys with an exactitude within fractions of millimeters. The human body can combine strength, stamina, and balance with infinite precision. No robot ever developed can duplicate any of these complex activities.

Just based on these observations alone, there can be no doubt. We are designed to move. And throughout most of our history, we've had to do that just to survive. Then along came the twentieth century and our inventive brains outpaced our bodies. We became focused on making machines to do the things we didn't want to do. And that freed us up to create jobs that are more brain-based than physical—the rise of the office job that has absorbed much of the workforce.

Unfortunately, our biology hasn't changed. We are still physical beings and just like the animals, if we don't move, we deteriorate. Most likely we would die as well, if it weren't for today's technology and medical intervention. This is not idle speculation. People on a prolonged flight, who sit for as long as seventeen hours or more, are at risk of developing deep vein thrombosis (blood clot in a large vein) because of lack of movement. Astronauts who spend weeks in zero gravity have to exercise to avoid muscle loss. Elderly people who have lived mostly sedentary lives often have difficulty getting up out of chairs and climbing stairs and are subject to falls because of lack of balance. A person who has been bedridden for a long period of time has to engage in physical therapy to get completely well again.

The necessity of exercise may not seem obvious because over the decades we have come to accept our sedentary lifestyle as normal. Yet, it isn't normal in terms of what our bodies are designed for and how they work. And when I refer to *body*, I mean our whole being. Activity influences mind, and mind influences body. They work together, and there are consequences when we decide one is not as important as the other. Throughout most of human existence, a normal level of physical activity was much higher than it is now in our age of automation. Consequently, if we want to be healthy in both body and mind, we need to find some way to make up for all that lost activity.

THE BENEFITS OF MOVEMENT

Not everyone aspires to be an elite athlete. But everyone can benefit from some kind of movement. Here's a short list of those benefits:

- Muscular and skeletal fitness
- Flexibility
- Increased stamina
- Improved balance
- Better circulation
- Reduced pain
- Shape-shifting effects
- Increased mental sharpness
- A sense of well-being
- Defense against depression
- Lower blood pressure
- Burning up extra carbs that would otherwise be converted to fat
- Triggering hormones that help your metabolism function properly
- Potential to delay the aging process (physical and mental)

You can't get around it: physical activity is a key ingredient in good health.

My theory about exercise and aging:

There's plenty of evidence that people who get some kind of regular exercise—even if only walking—live longer and healthier lives. My thought is that toned muscles are a sign of youth and vigor. They indicate to your metabolism that you are actively engaged in living and that you can contribute to your tribe.

Becoming sedentary, on the other hand, is a signal that you're winding down. If you're going to sit on the couch all day like a mushroom and let your muscles turn to flab, your body metabolism is going to think, "Well, we're done here. Nothing more to do—time to wrap it up." Essentially, by staying fit and active as long as you can, you trick your body into thinking you are still young.

THE BARRIERS TO MOVEMENT

Unfortunately the term *exercise* carries a lot of baggage. Exercise implies an activity that takes a lot of concentrated effort:
- It requires special scheduling.
- It conjures up images of someone sweating it out in a gym, straining to keep up on a treadmill or grunting to lift heavy weights.
- It carries the no-pain, no-gain sound bite with it.

Consequently, it puts people off. Just the thought can elicit a groan, spawning the joke, "Whenever I get the urge to exercise, I just lie down until the feeling goes away."

Exercise, by itself, with no other purpose, is not natural. It was never needed until the twentieth century because just the daily tasks required for living kept people active and fit. Which brings me back to the issue at hand: in order to maintain a level of physical activity that at least keeps us reasonably healthy, we have to do something more than our current lifestyle requires. But it doesn't have to be extensive formal exercise. That's why I prefer to call this section the Battle of Activity and not the Battle of Exercise. Activity is much more inclusive. And there are lots of ways to boost your activity that can be enjoyable and inexpensive.

THE TYPES OF ACTIVITY YOUR BODY NEEDS

To become physically fit, your body needs to be challenged in two different ways: aerobic endurance and strength. And you can meet both those challenges through everyday, informal activities as well as more formal, scheduled activities.

I have devoted one section to everyday activities which contribute to both aerobic endurance and strength, one section specifically for scheduled aerobic activities, and one for scheduled activities for developing strength. I hope to convince you there are ways to work on them that aren't painful.

SETTING THE RIGHT GOALS

Listen to the fitness experts and you'll likely feel like you have to steel yourself mentally, get a thorough fitness evaluation as a baseline (at a fitness center) and then set major fitness goals with the help of a fitness coach. This is the exercise equivalent of a diet: you have to turn your life upside down to achieve artificial goals set for you by someone else. And that leads to yo-yo exercising: weekend warrior or exercise boot camp followed by burnout and long periods of no exercise with a ton of guilt. And then what do you do when you're finished? You have the same problem with fitness maintenance that you do with diet maintenance.

When I first had the opportunity to join a fitness club, I had one of those assessments myself. I was in my mid-fifties and my evaluation coach looked to be about twenty-two. She took me through the paces. First we measured weight and body mass index (BMI), and I scored 32 percent body fat even though I'd been working out aerobically for years. That was my first disappointment because the recommended score for women is around 24 percent. I didn't do too badly with the cardio test, but when it came to strength I might as well have been a jellyfish. She had me lie down on a mat, gave me a metal bar, and asked me to raise it up as many times as I could (bench press) for a minute. What a joke! It weighed thirty pounds and I couldn't even lift it once. I think on a scale of one to ten, I must have been a negative five.

With the evaluations out of the way, she proceeded to tell me she could create a fitness program for me that would get me from a 32 to 28 percent in five weeks. I couldn't help laughing, and I thought, *You and what miracle?* My diet was very healthy and I'd been exercising for many years already. Maybe, if I'd been twenty-five, it would've been possible, but not at fifty-four. I knew from experience that five weeks wouldn't get me anywhere near that goal unless I drastically modified my diet and worked out eight hours a day. You see, we're not all the same body type; some of us are just not easily made fit according to standards. The coach's unrealistic expectations discouraged me from signing up for her program.

I've since observed that most clubs/regimens/programs have similar fitness evaluations. They usually have tests measuring how many push-ups or sit-ups you can do per minute, and so on. But, I believe these are artificial means of fitness evaluation and do not assess your *fitness for living*. The fitness measures clubs use today may be well intentioned, but they only serve to create fitness programs that generate money for the club. There are plenty of other more meaningful measures of fitness for life.

Certainly, if your goal is to be an Olympic or professional athlete, it requires intense physical effort. But most of us have different life goals and we just want to be fit enough to support those goals and engage in activities we enjoy. Some days my physical goal is just to get out of bed. But I'm one of those people with a job that puts me in a chair in front of a computer every day—writing software or writing a book—so I am acutely aware of a need for some extra physical exertion. To remedy that I've developed some activity goals that I try to meet every day.

Physical activity needs to be put in proper perspective. Too much focus on getting fit can lead to an obsession, and obsession leads to burnout. When you're looking to make a lifelong change, that's the wrong approach. I want to be fit but it's not my only goal in life—it's not even my primary one.

BUT BEFORE YOU START: A CAUTION

My intention in this battle is to give you an overview of various types of physical activities in case you don't already have this information. Also to tell you my story: how I got started with activity, how my routines evolved, how I've dealt with adversity along the way, and how I won this battle.

I'm in no way qualified to advise you on what you should do or how you should do it; I can only describe what I've done myself. It's probably safe to suggest at least that you can go for a walk. However:

- You should always get clearance from your physician for more strenuous activity.
- If you're going to participate in any activity that requires a particular skill, you should get instruction from a professional.

While extreme exercise can be bad, moderate activity is not, and there are light activities that anyone can do, even in a chair. The bottom line is that there are more benefits from *moderate regular workouts* than from irregular extreme ones.

HOW TO APPROACH THIS BATTLE

This battle could be overwhelming if you tried to do everything at once. But that's not the idea. You don't have to start exercising like crazy. As a matter, of fact that would be the worst thing you could do. In the coming sections, I'll present ways you can gradually incorporate more activity into your life—activities that support both strength and aerobic endurance. And hopefully, ways that won't be so boring you'll want to quit. This section on The Battle of Activity contains a lot of information because I want you to see the possible *choices* you have. If you are already active you probably have a good idea about how to proceed. If not, don't worry. I suggest the following:

1) Read the section to get an overview.
2) Start by working a few of the Everyday Activities into your daily schedule.
3) Of the scheduled activities, tackle a little bit of aerobics first.
    o Decide if you want to do it on your own or join a gym.
    o Try adding ten–fifteen minutes of aerobic activity such as walking (outside or on a treadmill) three times a week.
    o Try increasing that amount of time or frequency.
    o Stick with this for a couple of months.
4) Begin some scheduled strength training—which can be as little as ten minutes twice a week.
    o Decide if you want to do it on your own or join a gym.
    o Either way, schedule a session with a trainer first (see the website for potential free or low-cost options).
    o Decide if you want to continue with the trainer or gym, or if you want to go solo.
5) Use a simple chart to monitor your progress. See samples in *Appendix B* or use the online workbook, Battle of Activity, Actions #14 and #24.

The goal is to do a little more each month until you feel you've reached the maximum time and effort your schedule will allow. No one can tell you exactly how much to do because everyone is different, depending on body type, age, fitness level, and many other factors. The end result is personal and subjective.

The Challenges

ESTABLISH A BASELINE

Action #1: Assess your life goals

When you have some quiet personal time, take a few minutes to think about your real goals in life. Are they physical, social, introspective, mental? Do you want to be a doctor, lawyer, parent, software developer, farmer, writer, actor, athlete, or one of the other seemingly infinite choices we have available to us today?

If they are physical, focusing on increasing your physical activity will be a top priority for you and you may already be working on it. If your goals are more social, introspective or mental, winning this battle will help you keep active enough to be healthy without making you feel like the activity is taking over your life.

Make a note of your goals in the online workbook or a personal journal (paper or electronic). They may change over time.

Action #2: Determine your physical status

There are three things you should do before you start ramping up your activity:
- Check with your physician.
- If possible, get an evaluation from a licensed physical therapist (not a fitness club)
- Write down any physical limitations you have.

Once you have this information you can increase your activity without causing yourself injury or other physical harm. Always work within your personal medical guidelines.

OVERCOME ACTIVITY BLOCKAGE

Action #3: Identify your biggest barriers

If you've been a yo-yo exerciser, you'll want to identify the barriers that make you quit so you can face them head on. You're probably already well aware of most of the common barriers: lack of motivation, lack of time, lack of time *for yourself,* lack of momentum, finding the right venue, lack of daylight hours, bad weather, physical limitations, fear of bad consequences—or maybe you just don't want to do it.

While occasionally there are times in our lives when these barriers are insurmountable, most of the time it's a matter of priority. If you think something is important enough you can find a way. Here are some suggestions.

Lack of motivation. Motivation comes from inside you, not from outside, and if you don't have it you might start to exercise but won't sustain it. We all want to live happy, healthy, long lives. Try to fully internalize the fact that we are physical beings, and for that to happen we need to move.

Lack of time. Everyone is short on time. However, I think the biggest problem is the *perception* that to become more fit you have to commit to a major workout every day, or at least five days a week. Get it into your head that this level of commitment is *not* required. Instead, understand that *something* is better than *nothing*. And the process of *resetting normal* is to start out with some small change you can manage, assimilate it into your normal, and move on from there. Just start with ten minutes, three days a week. Make it a habit. If nothing else, you'll have ten minutes of peace and quiet to yourself.

If your life is so jam-packed that you can't even find ten minutes three times a week then you have a different set of problems than this book is designed to help you with.

Lack of momentum. Think small. It takes a lot less effort to get the momentum up for a ten-minute walk or an aerobic warm-up than for a half-hour or hour-long workout. Once you get used to doing it and your body adjusts, you'll have the momentum to continue. It won't be that hard to bump it up later to fifteen minutes; that additional five minutes won't seem like much at all.

Finding the right location. The answer to this depends on what you prefer, what's convenient, and what it costs. Maybe you can partner with someone else at first and take a short walk with him or her. You can also take a walk around the local mall or a school playground or track if one is close by. There are lots of choices, and you don't have to make the same one every time. You can vary your place so you don't get bored.

Dealing with your geographical location. Where you live and the time of year will influence whether your activity is indoors or outdoors. It all depends on your tolerance for certain extremes. Living in Seattle I see lots of people walking, running, and cycling in terribly rainy weather: they've just adapted to those conditions. If you live in Arizona you may have the opposite problem; how to be active outdoors when the temperature is over 100. Sometimes indoor activity is the only sane choice.

Physical limitations. If you're wheelchair-bound, have had an injury, use a walker, have a disability that makes walking impossible, or you're a senior dealing with age-related problems, you can still engage in some kind of movement. Check with your physician and a physical therapist and I'm sure you'll get recommendations that will help. Consider chair-based activities.

Fear of bad consequences. Sometimes bad things happen to people when they exercise, but it's always when they overdo it. If you push yourself too hard you'll injure yourself, or you'll damage ligaments and joints in such a way that later in life you'll need surgery to fix them. Personally, I'm cautious and I try not to get carried away. I've had only a few minor injuries along the way because I play it safe.

I just don't want to do it. Apply a cost/benefit approach. Consider what will happen if you don't become active and compare it with the benefits if you do. There are not only health consequences for staying sedentary, there are financial ones—perhaps not now, but certainly in the future. Investing a very small amount of time now will help you avoid those. And don't forget that one of the nicest benefits is that people who are active and fit look better and younger.

For this Activity, review the above list of the most common barriers and determine if any apply to you. Write them down in the corresponding Action in the online workbook and add any other barriers you think are standing in your way of becoming more active.

Action #4: Determine how you can overcome your barriers

Next to each barrier in Action #3, write down potential ways you can get over or around them. If I-just-don't-want-do-it is in your list, be sure to do that cost/benefit analysis. Be positive and creative. And think small steps—not solutions that mean you have to tackle a Major Project.

Action #5: Identify your biggest discouragements

Some people make it past the barriers above and then drop out because they get discouraged when they fail to meet common expectations. The best way to overcome the common discouragements is to set realistic expectations for yourself and turn off outside noise.

Not the expected weight loss. The biggest disservice that the experts have done is to associate exercise with weight loss, supported by the calories-in/calories-out formula. Just purge that concept from your mind. You might lose weight from exercise or you might not. But *it doesn't matter!* Whether you lose weight or not, you'll accrue all the benefits that come from regular physical activity. And that's what's important in the long term.

Not the expected body-shape changes. The best way to deflect disillusionment here is to accept the physical reality that your body has its own natural form and its own timeline for changing and if you want to get into *your* body's best shape, you'll need to make a lifetime commitment to physical fitness. All those commercials for fitness clubs, exercise machines, public service promotions, etc. that feature exercising models with Olympic-caliber athletic perfection? Ignore them. Just stop watching them. It isn't realistic to think we can look like they do. The main point of physical activity is to achieve a healthy level of fitness. If we can do that and maintain it, we will also look our best. And you can't do better than that.

Comparing yourself to the person next to you. If you're comparing your level of achievement to some randomly chosen person you know, remember that we're all different—physically, mentally, and in our life situations. Compare yourself only to yourself at another point in time. Just do what you can do and eventually the results will become evident.

You could always choose to engage in an activity by yourself, but if you enjoy class activity itself you'd be missing out. Besides just reminding yourself that it's ok if you're not the best, you can look for a beginner-friendly class. Some classes specify the level of expertise expected and if you don't think you fit, don't enroll. Better to start out at a lower level; you can always move up if it gets too easy. And it's better for your self-esteem.

Physical injury. It can be discouraging if you've done your best but still have done something wrong that caused an injury. Giving your body a workout is a learning experience. Do something wrong? Try to identify what it was, then back off for a while and try to avoid doing it again.

Some activities are more prone to causing injury than others. Probably the absolute safest activity is walking because it's something we all do in the normal course of our lives. But don't limit yourself, just try to be careful. Take the time to heal and gradually restart the activity. I've experienced a few injuries over the years, so I had to scale back and gradually start up again. It's always worked out positively for me in the long run. The benefits of regular, moderate physical activity will outweigh any minor injury if you're careful and conservative.

For this Activity, think about what has discouraged you in the past. What times, if any, did you start an activity and then quit because of something that discouraged you?

Make a list of things that discourage you most—situations most likely to make you quit.

Action #6: Make affirmations to overcome your discouragements

Positive affirmations are phrases you repeat to yourself to help you become what you want to be. They counter negative self-talk that rattles around in your head and keeps you down. Here are some positive affirmations to help you combat your discouragements. You can use these or you can make your own. If there are things that discourage you that aren't on this list, make *positive* statements to counter those things.

Not the expected weight loss
    My body will lose weight according to its own timeline.

Not the expected body-shape changes
    I respect and love the unique body that nature gave me.
    My body is amazing as it is.

Comparing yourself to the person next to you
   I am unique.
Physical injury
   I am careful and patient with my body.

Repeat your affirmations once or twice a day or whenever you feel discouraged.

SUPERCHARGE EVERYDAY ACTIVITY

If you are one of people in the workforce that has a physically demanding occupation, you can probably skip this section because you're already active all day long. Congratulations! You've completed this goal by default. But for the rest of us who have jobs with the physical requirements of a mushroom this is about ramping up everyday physical movements in little ways to help fill the activity void.

There is only one barrier to interfere with this goal: a lack of momentum. When you're not naturally active you have a *habit of inactivity* and you tend to think of ways to avoid moving your body. It's just hard to get going. But because there's only one barrier, it's a great place to start. Sneaking small physical challenges into your daily routine will kick-start that momentum and keep it going. These tiny activities aren't hard but the challenge is *remembering* to incorporate them.

Don't think just because they're mini-activities they couldn't possibly do any good. I've learned through experience that it doesn't take much to improve physical fitness. I've been through a couple of rounds of physical therapy where the restorative exercises took only ten minutes a day and yet fixed my problem completely in a couple of months. Small changes accumulate over time. As your muscles respond it will get easier.

Rules for these activities:
- *Do not* think of it in terms of burning calories toward weight loss.
- *Do* think of it as a way to develop better muscle tone, posture, and stamina.

The activities that follow have both aerobic and strength benefits.

Action #7: Add some mini-activities to your daily routine

We get so used to doing things the same way all the time, we miss opportunities to be active. Here's a list of a few to consider:

Take the stairs whenever you have the chance. It may seem like a pain but it does make a difference. I started by doing this at work a couple of times a week and gradually added more times. I had that opportunity because I worked on the third floor and the stairwell was right next to the elevator. I got an extra boost from it in the morning because I lugged a twenty-five-pound backpack and five-pound lunch pack to work every day. And doing it with that extra weight made me feel like a feather when I was going up the stairs without it. As I got more used to it, I made sure never to ask myself if I wanted to take the stairs or the elevator; I just took the stairs by default.

Of course, not every workplace offers that opportunity. Some are all on one level and others don't have stairs you can take, and if you work in a high-rise, you're not likely to hike up twenty or thirty stories. So maybe you can't do it at work. But there are other places to look. If you have a two-story house, use the stairs as often as you can. If you have several items to move from one floor to another, make two trips instead of one. If you're at the mall and stairs are available, take them instead of the escalator or elevator. I've been doing this for a long time and I'm amazed at how easy it is for me to sprint up the stairs now—and how great it feels to be able to.

Get up from your desk and walk around for a couple of minutes. Work can be mentally absorbing and it's easy to forget how long you've been sitting without moving much. I have heard from some experts that you should get up from your desk and stretch every ten minutes. I think this is completely unrealistic. Most desk jobs require concentration and, for me, even breaking every half hour or hour severely interrupted my workflow. I found it best to aim for a mid-morning and a mid-afternoon break; that's what seemed the most natural.

What things can you do on those short breaks?
- Visit the restroom.
- Get a drink of water/coffee/tea from the kitchen.
- Walk over to someone's office to ask a question (instead of asking via email).
- Walk around the periphery of the office.

- Take a brief walk outside around the block.
- Do a couple of pushups against your desk or other prop, or make a trip to the restroom and use the counter.
- Go up and down the stairwell a few times.

The important thing is just to get up more often and do something physical for five or ten minutes. It may not seem like much, but the accumulation of all these little things helps get your circulation going and develops your muscle tone. And you'll come to depend on it because it will help refresh both your body and your mind. Once I got used to taking that short activity break, I had no trouble remembering it. Now, my body reminds me: if I've been sitting for too long I feel fidgety, and the only way I can relieve that is to get up and do something physical. For other ideas, check out the book *Scared Sitless*, by Larry Swanson.

Park farther away from the store instead of wasting time, gas, and patience prowling for a space near the door. This is another case where time and/or weather is a deterrent. If it's convenient at the time, I will do it. If not I won't. But I don't beat myself up over it. At least I'll have that option on my radar and not dismiss it entirely. You may only be adding a few hundred steps, but walking is one of the best activities ever and your body will appreciate it.

Cook something from scratch. Time is short and we're all convenience-oriented. But pick one meal, maybe once a week, and try not to use all the common shortcuts. Examples:
- Grate your own cheese—this is great exercise for your arms.
- Chop the onions and celery by hand instead of a food processor.
- Slice your own lettuce or cabbage.
- Prepare a fresh vegetable like broccoli or carrots.
- Peel and slice your own potatoes for oven fries.

Just walking around the kitchen or standing while sautéing something keeps you off the couch and doing something physical. Don't get carried away and try to account for all the calories these activities might burn. Burning calories is not the point, but rather giving your body opportunities to move.

Action #8: Choose a mini-activity over standing or sitting still

There are plenty of times during the day when you're stuck in one spot, for instance waiting for the microwave to finish, or waiting for a bus, a person, or a meeting. Consider substituting a tiny activity instead of just standing or sitting in place. Below are some examples.

You can do them at your desk, standing in the kitchen, watching TV, waiting for the bus—whenever you happen to be at a standstill.

Stretch. Stretching is as good for you as any other form of activity. It relieves tension and promotes flexibility. And this is something you can do just about anytime in a matter of a minute or so.

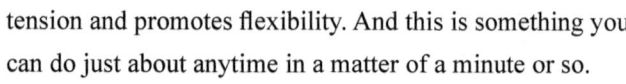

Practice balance. Whether you're heating up something for lunch at work or cooking something for dinner, while you're poised for that interminable microwave wait (which might be only a minute or two but seems like forever) there's one thing you can do that your colleagues probably won't even be notice. You can practice balancing on one foot. Balance is critical to physical fitness and this is an easy way to improve it. Just steady yourself, lift one foot off the floor and try to stay balanced on the other one for at least thirty seconds. Then switch to the other foot. I've been doing this for years and I don't think anyone's ever noticed—at least no one's ever said anything about it.

Do a couple of deep knee bends holding onto the counter. You can do this if you're in the restroom at work or when you're at home in the kitchen. Just hold onto the edge of the kitchen counter or sink, and bend your knees down then back up again. If you're not used to this kind of activity, protect your knees by starting with a shallow bend and just do it a couple of times. You can always increase the depth and the repetitions if you feel like it, but it's important to remember that this is not a heavy workout. It's only an activity to keep you moving instead of standing still.

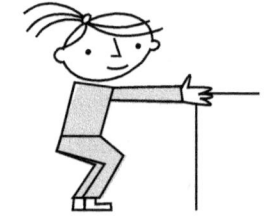

Do a couple of push-ups against the counter or wall. You can also do this if you're in the restroom at work or when you're at home in the kitchen. Simply put your hands on the counter, stand back a little bit and push away from the counter and back down.

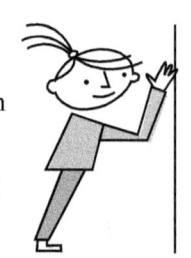

The farther back your feet, the more horizontal you'll be and the more work for your shoulders. But the idea is not to make this effort difficult—only to give your shoulders a bit of a workout and your body some physical activity.

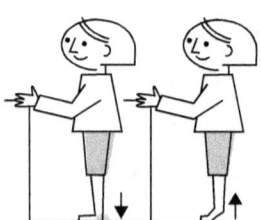

Heel raises. Try this anytime you have a minute or two and you're wearing comfortable shoes (or none). Hold onto something (counter, doorway or something similar) if you need to for balance, then raise yourself up on your toes. You can do this with both feet at the same time, then move to doing each foot separately. You get even more benefit if you do it on a stair, holding onto the railing. A couple of times is fine.

Do one or two jumping jacks. If you're somewhat ambitious, don't have any back or knee problems and do have a little space around you, try doing just two or three jumping jacks. Because I have back problems and jumping up and down puts a lot of compression on the lower spine, I have substituted a simulation: I do the usual arm motions, but just move one leg to the right or left, leaving the other stationary—no jumping involved.

Invent your own arm exercises. If you have a few minutes when you're just standing around and you're not out in public, try inventing a simple sequence of arm movements. Stretch your arms up, to the side, or down in any way that seems comfortable. You can enhance this by adding some weight with whatever is handy: a briefcase, a book ... use your ingenuity.

Action #9: Find fun ways to be active

Challenge your kids to a hand-wrestling match. If you have kids, try a couple of rounds of hand wrestling. I'm not suggesting anything competitive, just a little mild resistance training here and there. Depending on their age, you can let them win or not. And you both might get a laugh out of it—which is also good for your health.

Gardening, anyone? Not everyone enjoys gardening or has the time for it, but if you do, this is a great activity to keep you physically busy. The walking, stretching, bending, and lifting that's required—as long as you're careful—are good for you. And, if you're raising edibles, you get fresh food.

Yardwork. Rake leaves or mow the lawn.

Dancing. Put on music and dance around the room.

Family sports. Badminton, lawn darts, croquet, etc.

Juggling. A plus for coordination.

Action #10: Gradually increase your daily activity level

Gradually increase your activity level until you're active for much of your day. The total amount of activity is difficult to quantify—you shouldn't have to track it—but you should feel like you're not sitting, lying, or standing around for hours at a time without inserting some kind of minor movements into that space. This kind of activity is not about burning calories to lose weight. It's about developing and maintaining muscle tone and flexibility and reaping all the benefits that come from that.

If you want, you can list the benefits you feel from your added activity.

You'll find that as you get fitter, you'll enjoy it more and your desire to do it will increase. When you reach what you feel is a comfortable level, try to maintain it, but vary your activities so you don't get bored.

INCREASE AEROBIC ACTIVITY

The Context

What is aerobic activity?

An aerobic activity is one that requires oxygen, which means expending the kind of energy that requires your heart rate and your breathing to increase. Walking, running and dancing are all classic examples of aerobic activity. This is a little more formal than everyday activity because you need to specifically make time for it—probably the reason most of us don't get enough.

Benefits of aerobic activity

Aerobic activity develops the efficiency of your heart, circulatory system, and lungs, giving you endurance. In terms of everyday living, if you engage in regular aerobic activity you'll be able to walk longer, farther, and up stairs and hills without getting out of breath. You'll develop the momentum to keep you moving and off the couch because it won't take that much effort to get up. In essence, it will help reset your normal to the default of *active* rather than *inactive*.

Theory. I also have a theory about how aerobic activity might help your mental processes as you age. It stems from a child development theory that was prevalent when my kids were little. Back then we were encouraged to make sure that our babies learned to crawl before they walked. At the time it was thought that the alternating arm and leg movements involved in crawling helped develop the brain in a way that supported language skills. Now I don't know if this was ever proved, but in my theory I ask if it's possible that as we age, engaging in aerobic activity—especially activities that involve lots of different steps, like the variety you would find in dancing or step aerobics—might improve cognitive functions in the same way. Certainly, learning a dance routine requires memorization, coordination, and balance. That alone speaks well for this type of activity.

What I've done over the years

I didn't seriously start any kind of exercise regimen until I was 39. At that point I just adopted a mindset that it was time to do something about getting my body into shape. The path of least resistance? Walking. I started out walking around one block once a day and gradually, over a year's time, worked up to a couple of miles. A few years later I added low-impact step aerobics that I could do at home in any weather. It wasn't until about fifteen years later that I tried a fitness club and got to use the treadmill and elliptical machine. A couple of years after that I dropped out of the club experience and bought my own treadmill. Basically, those are the only aerobic activities I've engaged in because they are inexpensive and convenient.

What I learned that might help you

Don't overdo it. Over the last fifteen years I've learned that the best balance for me is a routine that includes some kind of aerobic activity three to five times a week. I have tried six days a week and it was too much—your body needs a rest. My advice: just do what you're comfortable with because if you overdo it, you'll burn out and quit. Something is better than nothing.

Don't forget to breathe. Apparently, breathing adequately for aerobic activity is not a built-in function. I never thought much about it until I read that the aerobic in aerobics means oxygen and that you won't get the full benefit from it if you don't breathe correctly[15]. I realized then that I tended to alternate between barely breathing and gasping to catch up. The best strategy is to set a pace based on your movement. For example, if you're walking, breathe in then out every two steps. I had to consciously practice that.

How to deal with interruptions. There have been times that I had to stop the aerobics for months due to schedule constraints or just plain lack of stamina (for unknown reasons). Occasionally, after these lapses I had to go all the way back to the warm-up level. But that turned out to be ok—I learned to be patient with myself, and just doing what I could eventually paid off because every time I had to retreat, it took less time to get back up to speed.

Don't feel compelled to extremes. There seems to be a lot of pressure today to go out, start running, and train for a marathon. But not all of us are built for that, and we risk potential injury both in the present and later in life. You don't have to run to get physically fit. Walking is good enough. And if you have the ability, walking uphill or setting a high incline on the treadmill goes a long way toward improving physical fitness; you don't have to obsess over speed. Activities like skiing, skating, swimming, tennis and other similar sports fall into the same category. If you like them and you feel you won't risk injury, great. If not, do what you can.

Benefits I experienced

I have to face reality: I'm seventy-plus years old and have arthritis, and my back discs don't have much padding between them anymore. So I don't expect to be jumping around like a gazelle; I just want to be able to function with minimal or no pain as I go about normal daily tasks. Regular aerobic activity has done this for me. When I get up in the morning my joints are stiff and sore, but after a ten-minute aerobic warm-up I'm pretty good. Then, after a full workout, I'm ready for the day. No pain medication needed.

Regular aerobic activity has also stabilized my back problems. Physical therapy for a major pinched nerve episode taught me that walking is one of the best activities for fixing and preventing back pain. Over the years, a regular, persistent walking schedule has kept me from recurring episodes.

I have more stamina than I did twenty years ago. I can sprint up and down stairs. I can walk up and down hills. I can walk around all day shopping. I have energy to spare. I can cook all day or work in the yard for hours. I have no trouble getting up out of a chair or the car or up off the floor. And it feels good to be able to do those things.

Don't fret about the details

When should you work out? There have been various studies that try to determine the best time of day to do exercise. I say it doesn't matter, as long as you do it. I prefer to do mine in the morning for two reasons: 1) I'm a morning person—I do not have the energy to exercise in the evening and 2) Once I've done it, nothing can take it away from me. If I wait until later in the day, something will invariably crop up and derail my best intentions. However, I know people who do much better later in the day. Some even prefer nine or ten at night. So, the answer to this question is: exercise whenever you feel most comfortable and you'll actually do it. All the noise around what time of day is most effective? Forget it, just do it.

How often and for how long? If you're not used to doing any of these activities on a regular basis, start with ten minutes, three times a week. Most of the guidelines for aerobic exercise, such as those from the American Heart Association, decree that you should work out for at least thirty minutes three times a week, but you don't have to do that to start with. You can get there eventually, at your own pace, by adding a few minutes when you feel you're ready. And don't feel guilty about taking your time. Remember, you're building a lifetime habit a little at a time; you're not training for the Olympics.

What about intensity? Intensity is a relative concept and there are various ways to measure it. One way is to monitor your pulse and get it up to the level recommended for aerobic exercise for your age. Another is perceived effort, where you learn to judge when you've reached your upper limit for the day. I like the latter method of measurement because everyone has good days and bad ones—a lot depends on your stress level, how much rest you've had, what you've had to eat, and probably a bunch of factors we aren't aware of yet. Occasionally I'll use a pulse monitor for safety, and I've observed that my average pulse can vary as much as ten points for the same workout from one day to another. I've never been able to determine what causes that difference, so I've decided it doesn't matter. I just do what I can without taking too much of a risk.

Based on recent studies, some experts say that short bursts of intense exercise are more beneficial than longer, slower ones. But how many times have the studies flip-flopped? One month it's short bursts and the next month the reverse. In my mind, it's micromanagement and second-guessing, so just go with what feels like it works. This is a learning experience. Start with what you're comfortable, with and you can always ramp it up a little at a time as your body adjusts.

What about measuring calories and carbs via the machines? If you're using a treadmill, an exercise bike, an elliptical machine, or some other electronic device, it's likely that it has the capability to measure your pulse, calories and carbs and to alert you to when you're in the so-called fat-burning range. I've learned never to take these measurements—which I call "treadmill math"—literally because all those calculations are based on whatever algorithms are built into the machine's program. It has no way of measuring what's actually going on inside your body. And setting your workout goals based on these statistics risks getting sucked into the kind of thinking where you figure if you've burned 400 calories, you've earned the right to have two donuts. Relative values are more important than absolute values. Just try to do a little more this month than last month.

What about interruptions? No matter what you plan for your exercise program, there are going to be interruptions. Vacations, holidays, illness, injury, daylight savings time, business trips, even lack of sleep. But that's ok. Sometimes you can compensate but sometimes you just need to back off and start up again. I've done this many times. But I keep on going because I feel much better overall when I've done some aerobic activity than when I haven't.

Now that I've reset my normal to an active state, on vacations and holidays I intuitively look for ways to be active. I've got nothing against sitting on the beach in the sun for a while or relaxing in a cafe, and I do some of that. But overall I prefer walking around, checking out the scenery, taking pictures—anything that gets me moving. And my holidays are active as well. Whether I'm home or visiting family, I'll be cooking and cleaning and shopping with everyone else. But if, despite everything, your time away from home is more sedentary, just go back to your normal aerobic schedule when you get home and you'll catch up quickly.

Back off when you're sick or injured and give your body time to recuperate. Because I monitor my blood pressure and pulse regularly, I've observed that both these measurements can be significantly higher after an illness so I may not engage in any exercise for several days or even a week. But as soon as I feel up to it, I will restart slowly—maybe just fifteen minutes' worth. I think it's important to get moving, as that helps with the healing, but I don't feel compelled to make up for lost time. Even if you need to cut way back at first, it doesn't take that long to get back to normal.

Action #11: Decide what, where, and when

The aerobic activities I chose were rather limited because I always went with what was most convenient and inexpensive, which was walking and step aerobics. With those, I can do as many or as few minutes as I feel like, and I can vary the aerobics workout by buying another DVD or downloading a routine from the internet. But there are many other possibilities. Aerobic activities include anything that gets you breathing more than normal, even regularly climbing stairs. Choose something you like that is as convenient as possible because if doesn't meet both these criteria you aren't going to stick with it.

Also consider your skill level and the expense. You don't need training or any equipment at all (other than a good pair of walking shoes) to go for a walk, but if you're going skiing you need to know what you're doing, and you need to invest in the proper equipment.

It's a good idea to have some variety too. Not just because it helps keep you from getting bored, but because each one of these activities uses different muscle groups. I got a free exercise bike from a friend and I expected it would be easy for me since I have so many years of experience with walking and aerobics. Big surprise: it was not easy at all. The same exercise doesn't even transfer from one environment to the next; if I've been walking mostly on the treadmill during the winter, my first outside-in-the-real-world walk will leave me with sore back muscles in places I would never think are involved in walking.

Some people like the idea of making exercise what I call a Major Project, but for those of us who don't have the time or the inclination for that level of effort, that's ok. There are plenty of ways to fit it in that don't take a huge amount of either time or money. The operative word is *sustainable*: you have to be able to incorporate your aerobic activity as part of your normal behavior, and if your workout is exhaustive that's not going to happen. So pick an activity that's both enjoyable and sustainable. One of the reasons I'm such a big proponent of walking—at least at first—is that it takes the least amount of time and money. You could think of walking as a gateway exercise: once you get started with it you may feel so good you'll want to try something else.

To get started, here are some suggestions:

Walk	Cycle	Jog	Run	Aerobics
Golf	Dance	Treadmill	Elliptical	Stepper
Tennis	Swim	Row	Ski	Snowboard
Rollerblade	Ice skate	Snowshoe	Hike	Team sports

Watch out for trendy workouts. There is always someone out there coming up with new workout ideas. And this is not a bad thing. If you think you'll enjoy one of them and it fits into your schedule, try it. Just be aware that if you're not in top shape already, injury is more of a risk. Make sure you start at a beginner level and learn what those risks are. The sports medicine business is booming these days, filled with people who have overestimated what their body is capable of handling.

Some of the more popular trendy workouts of late are Zumba, Crossfit, and kickstart or boot camp programs. The latter are patterned after military boot camp indoctrinations and based on getting you started with extreme physical exercises, none of which are sustainable unless you are an exercise fanatic. If you enjoy that kind of group activity and it's convenient, then try it. Just be cautious so you don't do more than you should and if you feel yourself getting tired of it, switch to something else.

The next step is to decide *where* you want to do your routine: at a fitness center or on your own.

And finally, decide when. It's easier to keep a regular schedule if you choose the same time each day, but if you can't find a common time, a specific time one day, and another specific time another day will work. The important thing is to choose one that is convenient enough to stick to.

If you're social, you might find it more interesting and fun to do these activities with a partner, or various partners—say, one for walking the neighborhood and one for the gym. In which case, all of the *what, where,* and *when* decisions would depend on a consensus with the partner.

Action #12: Get started with the minimum: ten minutes, three times a week

This Action is straightforward: once you have chosen an activity, time and place, just start doing it regularly. You don't need to track your intensity or try to figure out how many calories or carbs or fat you might have burned. This activity is not about losing weight—it's about starting a habit with which, over time, you can develop your stamina and all the other health benefits that come from that.

Action #13: Apply your first increase

Give yourself two to four weeks to make ten minutes, three times a week a habit. Then increase the time to fifteen minutes, three times a week.

Action #14 (optional): Sample aerobics tracking chart

If you want to keep track of your progress, a simple activity log will suffice. See a sample in *Appendix B*: Sample Aerobics Tracking Chart or use the online workbook, Battle of Activity, Action #14

Action #15: Apply gradual increases

Give yourself two to four weeks to make fifteen minutes, three times a week a habit you can keep. Then increase the minutes—five minutes at a time—until you reach your comfortable max (see the next Action). I suggest limiting the aerobics days to three because you should leave the other two days for developing strength. If you're using a chart, log your increases there.

Action #16: Decide when to level off

It's a good idea to aim long-term for a minimum of thirty minutes, three times a week. Obviously, you can do more if you have the time but don't try to increase it so much that it becomes a burden and you're tempted to quit. Thirty minutes is adequate. One hour would be awesome! The goal is to get so comfortable with whatever time you devote to this activity that you miss it when you can't do it. Then basically just keep doing it.

INCREASE YOUR STRENGTH

The Context

Strength training used to elicit visions of heavy weights, pain, and sweaty bodies but today none of those need apply if you don't want them to. I quickly discovered that you don't have to work at it two hours a day to improve your fitness; it's surprising how little time and effort it takes to make a big difference.

Benefits of strength training—why should you do it?

The benefits of becoming even a little stronger are obvious if you give it some thought. Strength training for the average person is about making everyday activities like walking, bending, lifting and going up and down stairs easier. When your muscles are strong you have a better sense and control of your balance, which means less risk of injury from a fall.

Here is a partial list of benefits. Strength training:
- Increases strength.
- Helps you stand taller and have better posture.
- Increases flexibility (from the stretches).
- Improves your sense of balance.
- Increases stamina.
- Protects you from injury.
- Counteracts shoulder and neck problems that a desk job inflicts.
- Helps with aerobics—muscles are able to do more with less effort.
- Is a shape-shifter—muscle can replace fat, reducing the jiggle factor.
- Increases skeletal strength.
- Helps keep muscle tone for better mobility as you age.

Strength exercise is especially important today because many of us sit so much commuting, working at a desk in front of a computer, or engaged in other sedentary activity that our muscles rarely get challenged in any way that would keep them from deteriorating.

What I've done over the years

My strength-training history is much shorter than my aerobic history. My work with weights didn't start until I joined a fitness club in 2002. The membership included one session with a trainer to explain how to use the equipment safely, and later I paid for a couple of private sessions. I learned the basics and have stuck with that—I don't do anything extreme—and that has served me well.

The essence of strength training is using resistance (weights or resistance bands) to challenge various muscle groups by repeating defined motions with varying weights or resistance. To develop strength, you start with low weight/resistance and a small number of repetitions and gradually increase both.

My modus operandi. Not wishing to risk injury, my approach was to try to work with my body, not against it. That meant getting very comfortable with one level of an exercise before increasing either the number of repetitions or the weight. Sometimes that would take a month or even more. I just worked at one level until it started to feel easy, then I upped it slightly. I never increased both the repetitions and the weight at the same time. As a matter of fact, when I increased the weight, I dropped the number of repetitions and worked my way up again.

Things I learned along the way

It doesn't take much. I'm always amazed at how little work it takes to improve. The best example of this comes from my introductory weight-machine tour. The trainer had me try the bicep curl machine at the lowest level of resistance. For this machine, you fit your arm into a support and then, grasping a handle, bend your arm at the elbow and pull the handle toward your shoulder. I could do it five times with my right arm. But when I tried the left arm the first pull set off a pain alarm. I stopped, thinking "Oops—that's not good!" Not wanting to give up, I thought I would try—gently—to improve it.

What I did was use my right arm to help the left one do the pull (right arm pushed while left arm pulled), going through the motions but making sure not to pull hard enough to trigger the pain. I did this only five times, twice a week for two weeks. Then I tried it with the left arm alone and voila! I could do it a couple of times with no pain. That's all it took to fix that problem: five times, twice a week for two weeks.

Similarly, I found that it took very few weight exercises to wake up my muscles and improve my fitness overall. With weights, sometimes less is more. I found that if I tried increasing the weights too fast, my progress actually slowed.

Be patient—progress is uneven. I learned to be patient with myself (for the most part). As I tracked my progress I observed that I could struggle along at one level for a long time, feeling like it never got any easier. Then—bingo—one day it suddenly did, and that's when I advanced to the next level. I also found that I didn't have to worry about a week or two vacation from weight training. As a matter of fact, frequently, coming back from a one-week hiatus, the exercises were easier. Sometimes your body just needs a break.

Watch out for the stretches. I learned to be gentle with the stretches, especially with any stretch that involved the lower back. Occasional discomfort after a workout was usually caused by overdoing a stretch, not the actual strength exercise itself.

It's important to set the right goals. There were times when I got overly enthusiastic about achieving a higher level of a particular exercise, I caused a minor injury. It's easy to fixate on the wrong things. For instance, starting with wall push-ups, I tried for at least five years to gradually work up to doing a floor push-up. But every time I attempted the real thing, I managed to injure a shoulder. I have since abandoned this goal, substituting planks instead, which is something I learned in my last session with physical therapy. My advice: unless you have professional coaching, don't try to emulate the super-fit people you see in videos. Listen to your body's feedback instead.

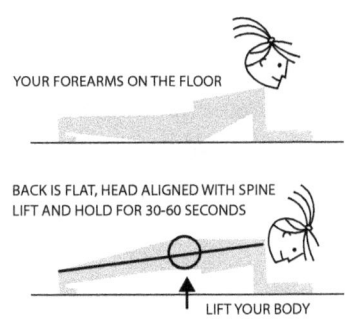

YOUR FOREARMS ON THE FLOOR

BACK IS FLAT, HEAD ALIGNED WITH SPINE
LIFT AND HOLD FOR 30-60 SECONDS

LIFT YOUR BODY

Know when to get professional advice. I'm not sure why I got so obsessed with the push-up goal in the first place. Now I think that if I really wanted to pursue it, it's one of those things for which I should seek the advice of a professional trainer. Maybe it's not even appropriate for someone my age and body type. If you're having a hard time with a particular exercise, either you're doing it wrong or you shouldn't be doing it at all. That's the time to check with a trainer.

What kinds of things can you do?

I'm sure there are more ways to engage in strength training than I know about so I can only list those that I am somewhat familiar with.
- Machine weights (at a gym or with a home unit)
- Free weights (at a gym or at home)
- Resistance bands (at a gym or at home)
- Pilates (at a Pilates studio)

Anything done at a gym or studio is going to take more time and money, but you'll get instruction and support if you want it. If you choose to buy a home unit, you need to get good advice because they can be expensive. Some are easy to use and effective, and some can be a waste of money. One advantage of doing free-weight or resistance-band work at home is that you don't have to buy everything at once. When I started I didn't know how heavy a weight I would advance to, so I didn't want to buy a full set. I just bought a couple of two-pound and five-pound weights, and it wasn't until months later that I felt I needed to get anything heavier. Resistance bands are much less expensive. Another advantage is that you can keep them handy and do a little workout while you're watching TV.

If your mobility is limited, there are even gym chairs on the market, designed with resistance bands so that you can complete a pretty good routine sitting in a chair. No matter what your age or physical condition, there's some sort of strength training you can try with professional help.

How should you start? Some internet jokes get repeated too much and aren't very funny, but I found the following one entertaining:

Advice for absolute beginners at weight training:
Begin by standing on a comfortable surface where you have plenty of room at each side.

With a 5-lb potato bag in each hand, extend your arms straight out from your sides and hold them there as long as you can.

Try to reach a full minute, and then relax.
Each day you'll find that you can hold this position for just a bit longer.

After a couple of weeks, move up to 10-lb potato bags.
Then try 50-lb potato bags and then eventually try to get to where you can lift one 100-lb potato bag in each hand and hold your arms straight for more than a full minute.
Finally ...
After you feel confident at that level, put one potato in each bag.

As silly as that is, there's a grain of good advice there: start out with light resistance and progress very gradually.

Don't fret the details

When should you do strength-training exercises? I'd suggest the same here as for aerobics. Choose a time that works for you, preferably the same time each day so it will be easier to remember.

How often do you need to do them and for how long? It doesn't take a lot to make a big difference. As a matter of fact, doing them too often can impede your progress. Per the trainer I had, twice a week is sufficient. As to how long, I started with ten to fifteen minutes, just like the aerobic activity. It's better to do a short time consistently than a long time erratically. Some people divide the workout based on muscle groups: one day they do upper-body and arm exercises and the next, focus on lower-body and legs.

What about interruptions? Just as with the aerobic activity, don't worry about interruptions. A couple of weeks of vacation from strength training won't set you back much, and if you've been sick, just ease back into the routine. If for some reason you have to stop for months, don't try to pick up where you left off; drop way back in repetitions and weight level and gradually build up again. For all the times I've had interruptions that long, I've never lost everything. The physical strength gained doesn't disappear unless, perhaps, you let it go for years.

Action #17: Honestly evaluate your level of strength fitness

If you've done strength training in the past you probably have a good idea of the level of difficulty you should start with. If you are a complete novice, however, you should get a *professional evaluation first*. Ask your healthcare provider if you can get a referral to a service such as physical therapy.

If you've decided that the best location for you is a gym, you can get an evaluation there. But keep in mind that the credentials of the evaluator might vary widely and the gym is in business to sell you services, a position that might influence the evaluation. I still think it's a good idea to get a baseline of your physical fitness from a medical professional.

Action #18: Decide on the best location for you

Based on your professional evaluation, convenience, cost, and comfort level with strength-building activities, decide whether you want to try this at home by yourself or in a gym or studio. Keep in mind that you can always change your mind later. But make sure that if you choose a gym, you can quit without penalty fees.

Action #19 (for home workouts): Decide on equipment

Decide if you want to invest in a home unit (which can be costly) or start with a few free weights or resistance bands.

Invest in a book that describes the workout you want. Do this even if you are purchasing a home unit. Your unit will come with some instructions, but probably not enough to be fully safe and effective. You could find instructional videos on YouTube but be sure to vet the credentials of the source. You don't want to risk injury by following an amateur.

I'm more familiar with basic free-weight exercises since that's what I use at home. Nevertheless, I am in no way qualified to teach others, so I'm not including any detailed instructions in this book. You don't need to start out with everything, but a well-rounded workout should eventually target all your major muscle groups. See *Appendix B*: Some Common Strength Activites or the online workbook, Battle of Activity, Action #20, for more detailed descriptions.

Here are two books you may find helpful. For more, see the Additional Reading section.

The Women's Health Big Book of 15-Minute Workouts (Yeager, Selene and
    Editors of Women's Health)
The Men's Health Big Book of 15-Minute Workouts (Yeager, Selene and
    Editors of Men's Health)

Action #20: Implement your home plan

Whether using a home-workout machine, resistance bands, or free weights, *I highly recommend first visiting a qualified trainer* to get some instruction and a workout plan that is tailored to you. The books are a great way to continue on your own, but form and safety are something best learned by someone who can guide you properly to start with.

At the very least, look for any of the following credentials:
- NASM (National Academy of Sports Medicine)
- ACE (American Council on Exercise)
- NACA (National Strength and Conditioning Association
- ACSM (American College of Sports Medicine)

Start with *only* ten minutes a day, two days a week.

There's a reason I specify only ten or fifteen minutes a day. It's because *before anything else*, you need to build the habit into your lifestyle. It's not the risk of overdoing it in terms of straining your muscles, but the risk of abandoning the activity altogether by making too large a commitment.

Obviously, in ten minutes you won't be able to do very many activities, but that's ok. If your fitness evaluator gave you a list of exercises to start with, do however many you can fit into that time. Don't try to do them all. Choose a couple for your upper body and a couple for your lower body. And start with a very light weight or none at all. When I began, I did many of these exercises without a weight until I thoroughly understood the position and the motions involved.

Action #21 (for gym or studio): Get familiar with the machines

If you want the standard strength training at a fitness club, there's a wide variety of types and manufacturers of exercise equipment, and not all fitness clubs use the same ones. Because of that, here's a partial list of the common ones (without pictures). You can look them up on the web or check with your local fitness club.

- Leg Press
- Leg Extension
- Seated Leg Curl
- Rowing machine
- Bicep Curl
- Triceps Extension
- Bench Press
- Shoulder Press
- Ab Crunch

Action #22: Implement your gym plan

At the very least, when you sign up for a fitness club, they should provide you with a basic tour of all the equipment and probably a set of recommended starter routines. Start with that. If you elect to pay for a personal trainer, they will create a plan for you with a variety of exercises tailored to your goals.

Either way, I strongly suggest you ask them for a very short beginner plan. I still recommend the ten minutes a day, two days a week commitment to start with. You might be tempted to stay longer, simply because you've taken the trouble to get there. However, the same principle applies here as for at home. The habit should come first. Overcommitment can lead to abandonment.

Action #23 (for Pilates): Enroll in a Foundation class

If you select Pilates for your strength activity, I recommend signing up with a studio for basic instruction. There are two varieties: machine and mat. You might be tempted to try the mat variety on your own but don't—at least not as a beginner. Pilates targets some specific muscle groups that most of us are not used to using and which can be difficult to identify by looking at pictures in a book or watching a video. I thought I knew something about Pilates from a video I worked with years ago, but after recently attending a Foundation class, I found out I was doing the basic moves wrong. It takes a trained instructor to watch you and correct your movements. A qualified studio will explain both the mat and machine varieties to you and get you started.

Pilates classes will be a standard length and require you to start at a foundation level and gradually increase your expertise under supervision, so my ten minutes a day, two times a week recommendation doesn't apply. If you choose this method, make sure you can meet the time requirement.

Action #24: Gradually increase your strength activities

Once you can regularly execute a routine ten or fifteen minutes a day, two days a week for two to four weeks and feel comfortable with that, then extend it five minutes longer, two days a week.

There are two ways to increase your strength activity:

1) Increase the number of repetitions for each exercise.
2) Increase the weight (or switch to a higher resistance band).

A reasonable, safe way to progress is to work up to ten repetitions for each exercise and feel comfortable with that. Then increase the weight slightly and drop the repetitions down to five. But take your time and don't increase the weights or repetitions too fast. I add only one repetition at a time and increase the weight by the smallest possible increment, and I arrive at my goal without strain or injury.

Consider using a chart to help you track your progress. See *Appendix B: Sample Strength Training Tracking Chart* or the online workbook, Battle of Activity, Action #24, for a sample.

GET ENOUGH SLEEP

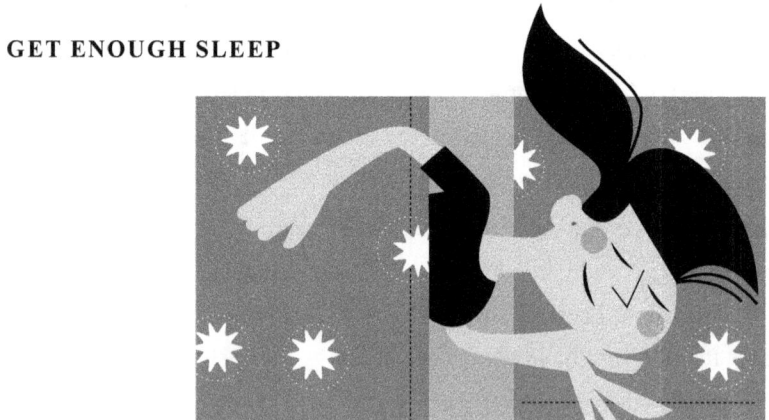

The Context

You might wonder why I have a section on sleep in the Battle of Activity. Just think of rest and sleep as activity in reverse. You can't ramp up your activity level much if you are rest- or sleep-deprived. Exhaustion will have just as negative an effect on your physical activity as it does on your appetite and food cravings.

Why sleep is so important

The news media frequently features studies on sleep. The results of these studies all seem to be the same: lack of sleep has all kinds of bad effects, such as decreased mental alertness, weight gain, and higher risk for cancer and heart disease. While I do appreciate the scientific curiosity and the desire to prove the benefits of sleep, my personal reaction is, "Duh."

Really, it seems obvious that when I'm sleepy my body is telling me it needs down time and when I get a good night's sleep I feel much better and I can work more efficiently. We get sleepy for a reason: our body needs time to repair itself, and to do that it needs not to have to focus energy on the physical demands of everyday life. When we sleep, our body needs only to maintain basic functions like heartbeat and breathing and can devote its resources to maintenance, repair, and probably a zillion other things we haven't discovered yet.

This is not a book about sleep, but a lack of sleep has a major impact on our ability to function efficiently and effectively and balance our appetite. If I try to solve a particularly difficult algorithm for a computer program at the end of the day when I'm tired, it never goes well. If I do it when I'm well rested, it's much easier. I get cravings for sweet foods when I'm exhausted but not when I'm well rested.

Your body has to keep going whether you allow it to sleep or not. My unscientific conclusion is that when it's rested, it's content to use its normal sources of energy. But when it's in sleep-deprivation mode, it demands quick energy—the kind that only sugar or refined processed foods provide.

Barriers for rest and sleep

Unfortunately, as much as we need sleep, there are too many modern reasons we can't always get it. While centuries ago candles provided light at night, most people went to sleep when it got dark and woke up at sunup. Today we have a 24/7 society with plenty of distractions to keep us from sleeping enough.

Stress and worry are probably the number-one reason behind lack of sleep. Work is another. Gone are the days of the 8 to 5 job—too many jobs now require that we be available all the time, even in the middle of the night. Technology certainly plays a major part. The internet is available all the time on a laptop, a tablet, or a phone. There are video games to play, on-demand movies to watch, and music to listen to, plus Facebook, Twitter, and a host of other social media distractions. I can't begin to list everything. And the problem is that they're all tempting and much more fun than sleeping, so it's easy to skip the sleep.

Common solutions

There are a number of natural ways to help you relax enough to get the sleep you need (including turning off the tech gadgets, controlled breathing, and meditation), but more and more people are resorting to taking sleeping pills to get their downtime because it's easier.

There's also a flood of technological approaches. I say approaches instead of solutions because they focus more on generating data about the problem than fixing it. Smart phone apps and other gadgets will track your breathing, pulse and sleep attributes. Sleep Number released a bed in 2014 that they call "Sleep IQ", which monitors your sleep and gives you a report on how you did for the night. I don't see how all that information is supposed to help me sleep better; I think I'd just worry more every time my statistics showed I didn't sleep well.

Sleep and weight

This is not a book about how to get sleep. However, I hope to convince you that you should take sleep seriously. Lack of it will negatively affect your performance, both mental and physical, and your appetite. It will also affect your attempt to reset normal.

I found out firsthand how lack of sleep leads to craving refined carbohydrates. I used to rise at 4:30 a.m. to get in my workout early. One of those mornings I woke up especially tired with a craving for a cinnamon roll. As I lay there thinking about it, I could envision what my day would look like if I got up as usual: I would work out, go to work, eat a large cinnamon roll, get hungrier, eat a large lunch with a cookie for dessert, and it would go downhill from there. It would not end well. So I went back to sleep, and when I woke up three hours later, voilà! Cinnamon roll craving completely gone—and the rest of my day was great.

The bottom line: is if you're not getting enough sleep, try to figure out why and find a solution. It may just be that if you snooze, you lose—weight, that is.

If you think you get enough sleep, feel free to skip the next set of Actions. If not, consider doing them; they don't take long.

Action #25: Evaluate the quality of your rest

Ask yourself the following:
- Do you have reasonably regular sleep hours? If not, why not? Is it family or work demands, electronic device addiction, or something else?
- Do you sleep well? If not, what is it that interferes with your sleep? Is it anxiety, worry, financial problems, thinking about work, physical pain, or something else?
- Do you feel sleep deprived (sometimes or all the time)? If so, are there particular days of the week that you become exhausted?

Action #26: Track your sleep/activity/eating patterns

Consider keeping a log of your sleep patterns for a couple of weeks, including date/time, type of day (work or time off), state of rest (rested, exhausted, etc.), state of hunger, food cravings, and energy level.

Here's a brief outline:
- Date and day of the week
- Work day or day off?
- Your state of rest:
    - o Well rested, wide awake
    - o Moderately tired
    - o Exhausted—it's an effort just to stay awake
- Are you very hungry?
- What foods do you crave, if any?
- Your energy level
    - o Energetic—feel like being active
    - o Lethargic—feel like sitting or sleeping

Action #27: Analyze your sleep/activity/eating patterns

Look over your tracking information. I doubt if you felt well rested and energetic 100 percent of your waking hours, and I hope you didn't feel exhausted 100 percent of the time. Most likely you experienced a mix of these states so you'll be able to correlate your state of rest with your activity/eating patterns. I found the following:
- When I was well rested: I wasn't hungry all the time and had no particular food cravings, and I felt inclined to be active.
- When I was exhausted: I felt like snacking all the time and craved sweet, highly refined foods—the kind that provide quick energy. I was inclined to inactivity and felt it was an effort just to stay awake.

You may also able to see where in your schedule you're most well rested and when you're tired. For me, I found I was well rested Sunday through Wednesday, started to lose energy on Thursday, and was totally exhausted Friday and part of Saturday.

The point of this Action is to closely observe how a lack of sleep negatively affects your activity/eating patterns.

Action #28: Identify potential solutions

It may be that you can't do anything about your schedule that will allow you to sleep better, but you should at least *think* about finding ways to improve it. You don't have control over everything, but some things are under your control—for instance, the time you spend on your digital devices, watching TV, or reading.

If you are losing sleep because of anxiety and worry, try Action #29.

Action #29: Learn a relaxation technique

I fall asleep easily, but I frequently wake up around 2:00 a.m. and have much trouble getting back to sleep. I call this my "witching hour" because during this time all my normal anxieties and worries become hugely exaggerated; they're like ghosts rising out of the graves in a cemetery and coming to haunt me. A few years back, however, I found a relaxation technique that helps me drive away those ghosts and lets me get back to sleep quickly. The technique is called *autogenics*, and you can find out about it at the website ***guidetopsychology.com/autogen.htm***, as well as on the *Resetting Normal* website. It takes a little patience to learn, but it's not difficult and is well worth your time.

Some people find meditation and/or yoga helpful as well.

Measuring Success

Winning the Battle of Activity is important because resetting your normal to active instead of sedentary will help you win the battles to come: The Battles of Quality and Quantity.

Ten tips for keeping you motivated:
1) Keep reminding yourself that exercise is for your health—*not for weight loss*.
2) Identify your barriers and find the easiest way around them.
3) Be persistent. Think like the tortoise vs. the hare—slow and steady wins the race.

4) Don't compare yourself to the picture-perfect athletes in the commercials—be the best you can be, not the best someone else can be.
5) Don't get completely derailed by interruptions. It's not a crime to back off and start over again and again—you gain something from the exercise with every iteration.
6) Watch for burnout—if you get sick and tired of one activity, switch to something else.
7) If you reach a point where you just don't have the energy, back off for a while.
8) Beware of perfectionism—"Done is better than perfect."
9) Work with your body, not against it—gradually build on what you have.
10) The important thing is the commitment of time. Show up at your appointed time and do something.

Physical activity benefits you as a whole person. If your goal is to be able to do more fun things in your life, like traveling, or simply managing daily life with more joy and energy, better physical fitness will make that easier. If you're a person who likes to shop, think increased shopping stamina. If you're someone who enjoys some kind of sport, whether it's softball or soccer or fishing, regular physical activity will make you better. And even if you don't lose a single pound, you'll be healthier for being active on a daily basis.

Winning The Battle of Activity is as much a mental shift as a physical one. When you've truly won you'll look for ways to engage in physical activity rather than ways to avoid it. *When active becomes your normal, inactive becomes intolerable.* We will never be as active as our ancestors were, but whatever we can do to partially fill the gap will contribute to our overall health.

NOTES

CHAPTER 9
THE BATTLE OF QUALITY

The Context

The Battle of Quality is the battle to replace processed, faux foods with real, natural, high-quality foods. It's not about losing weight. This battle is about restoration and healing: giving your metabolism what it needs to be strong, to get rid of cravings. If you're even tempted to go back to diet thinking anywhere along the way, repeat the following mantra:

> If you go on a diet, you cannot guarantee that you'll lose a certain number of pounds every week because you do not have control of how your body responds to deprivation. However, you *do* have control over what you choose to eat and drink.

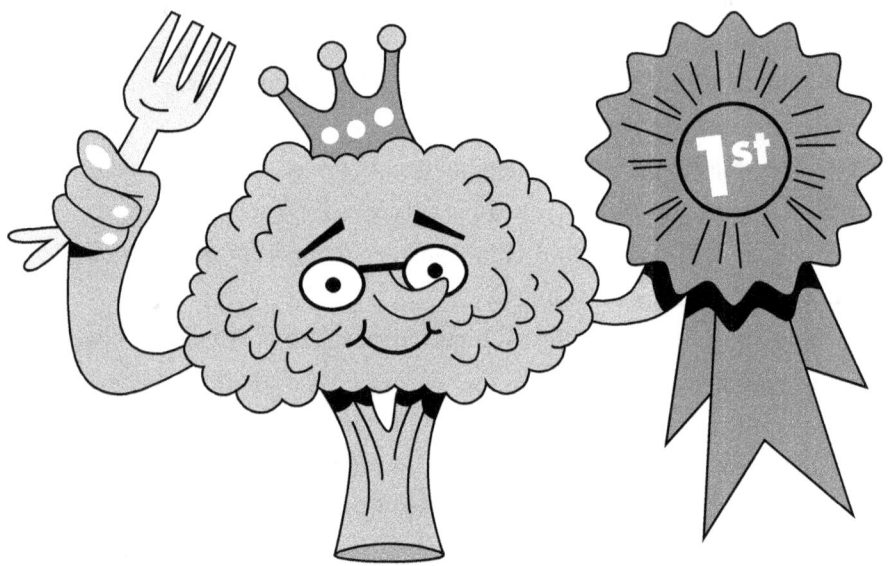

WHY WHOLE FOODS?

The whole-foods advantage

Whole foods give us the advantage of *quality*. What do I mean by that? When I talk about *quality* foods I'm referring to foods that have high values of nutritional elements in their natural form and satisfaction potential. This level of quality is important because *there is a direct relationship between quality and quantity*. When your metabolism is struggling to function with the junk it may have become used to, it sends the wrong signals to your appetite. Consuming foods of low quality fuels your appetite. Consuming foods of high quality satisfies your appetite.

You cannot win the last battle—the Battle of Quantity—for life until you have won the Battle of Quality. One of the failings of common diets is that they ask you to fight both of these battles at the same time, and that makes it difficult if not impossible to succeed. I specifically recommend that you do not engage in the Battle of Quantity until you can rate your Battle of Quality at least as a 60 percent win.

You are what you eat—literally

Part of *resetting normal* is gradually modifying what you like to eat, so it's important to understand why this is necessary and how it affects your general health. I'm sure you have heard the phrase "You are what you eat." I think everyone understands it at some level. You eat a hamburger or an apple or a muffin. Somewhere between your chin and your legs it gets liquefied and disassembled into some basic nutrients. Your body absorbs them, using them for energy to keep you moving and thinking. You keep on living, which wouldn't happen if you didn't eat.

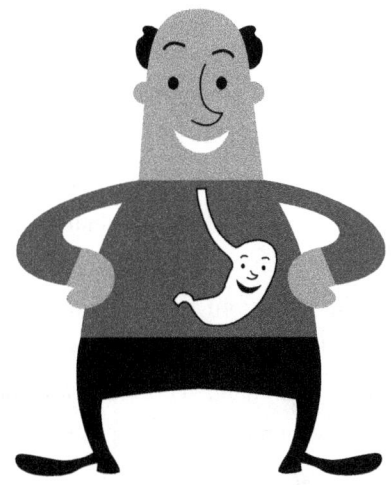

But because you keep on living as long as you eat *something*, you probably don't appreciate how much it matters *what* that something is. Or how it affects your quality of life. I always thought I did understand that, but it wasn't until I started learning more about the molecular biology of the human cell that I fully realized how literally true it is that we are what we eat. Food provides the stuff that supports all our bodily processes and which, over time, replaces every element and every cell in our bodies. If the food doesn't provide the right stuff then the processes don't work well and the replacements will be weak and ineffective.

Take a moment.

Close your eyes and breathe calmly and deeply. Let go of the tightness in your muscles. Feel your head and neck relax. Relax your shoulders, your back, your arms, your legs. Relax everything down to your feet. When you feel that your body is calm and quiet, open your eyes and read on.

What you probably weren't thinking about ...

If you took the moment described above, when you finished you probably felt like you weren't doing anything. But guess what? While you were sitting there feeling a state of relaxation, what was (and hopefully still is) going on inside your body was nothing less than a state of frenetic activity. Your heart was pumping, blood was rushing through your veins, thousands of chemical reactions were occurring in every cell of your body every fraction of a second, electrical activity was pulsing in your brain. And all this just to keep you alive while you were sitting there feeling like you were doing nothing.

What powers all that activity is chemistry. Every one of our cells is a little chemical factory. Your very existence depends on the chemical processes that happen inside the cells and between the cells. You take in food, which consists of molecules of various types. The food you take in gets processed by your digestive system and the resulting nutrients (minerals, proteins, enzymes, and a multitude of other kinds of molecules) are transferred into your bloodstream for dissemination throughout your body. The nutrients are used to produce energy, to build new cells, to repair damage by chemically reacting with each other, even to produce your thoughts. And this activity continues constantly until death. You are never the same physical entity today that you were yesterday, or one hour ago or even one second ago. Believe it or not, bit by bit you are completely replaced every couple of years.

And if the molecules you take in as food are not the type your body needs for this chemistry to happen correctly it could eventually cause disease and degeneration. That's why quality matters so much.

The package matters

I was in a supermarket not long ago and overheard a conversation between an older couple. The husband asked his wife, "How about apple juice? I can have that, can't I?" His wife responded, "Well, I guess so—it's fruit." Then he added, "Yeah, it'd be the same as eating an apple." And I wanted to scream, "Noooooooo! It's not the same!" But of course, I didn't. It isn't that apple juice is bad, but it's definitely not the same as eating a whole apple, and here's why.

Besides the fact that whole foods contain more of the nutrients we need to thrive, whole foods include something else we need: *the entire package*. The entire package includes all the *edible* parts of the food, not just an extraction of it—a whole peeled orange instead of just orange juice; the whole grain instead of just the starchy white endosperm; the whole egg instead of just the white.

Our body metabolism is so complex that science hasn't yet been able to reverse-engineer it. There's so much we don't understand. Not only haven't we identified all the nutrients the body needs, we also haven't identified all the interactions between all the nutrients. That's why we see studies that claim certain benefits for a particular minimum quantity of a nutrient and studies that contest that claim: it's a work in progress. Some elements we need in measurable quantities, like vitamin C or vitamin A. But others, like iodine or cobalt, we need in only trace (barely measurable) quantities. And it's very hard to figure out how they all work together.

In practical terms, the reason the package matters is that over the eons our *metabolic plumbing* has adapted to use foods as they mostly occur in nature. Natural, whole foods have all the co-factors (helper molecules) needed for your body to metabolize the nutrients effectively. They also have all the fiber your metabolism needs to regulate the flow of nutrients as it escorts the food from one end of you to the other. As soon as you start taking food apart and isolating particular components—as we have done in the last few centuries—you run the risk of eliminating something important.

When you get a package in the mail, you open it and throw away the box. Food is not like this. The food package is an integral part of the contents. The whole equals more than the sum of its parts, which is why we can't live off vitamin and mineral pills. Scientists can analyze a human body and identify all the molecules that it consists of. But there is no way they can gather all those molecules and assemble them into a human being. Nor can they assemble all the molecules that make up an orange into an actual orange with all its orange values. (Unless you live on the *Starship Enterprise*.)

Finally, the whole package tastes better and is more filling and enjoyable. I read an article about studies that are attempting to isolate the elements in wine and chocolate that seem to give us a health benefit—presumably so we could swallow the extracted element and avoid the calories of the real food. Sorry, but I don't really care. I'm not going to take a wine pill or a chocolate pill. I'd rather drink the wine and eat the chocolate any day and enjoy all the other benefits it supplies. And I've learned from *resetting normal* that I don't need to count calories anyway.

This is not to say that everything we eat has to be whole, but we certainly need much of it to be. Think, "The food, the whole food, and nothing but the food."

The satisfaction factor

Besides providing all the nutrients we need, real, whole foods provide appetite satisfaction. And they do this with two attributes: bulk and a balance of carbohydrates, protein and fat.

Bulk. A whole food has bulk, meaning it takes up space. It fills your stomach and makes you feel full in the short term. A big salad, two cups of broccoli, a couple slices of whole wheat bread, a bowl of beans and rice—each of these will take up a lot of space in your stomach and help you correctly decide when to stop eating. They also take a long time to digest so they keep you feeling full for a while.

Refined, processed foods do not fulfill this requirement, which is one of their dangers. These foods do not take up much space, making it easy to overeat. Take a piece of refined white bread and squish it into a ball in your hand—not much there. On the other hand, cut up a large apple into chunks and have about two cups. That's a lot of bulk, and it's going to take some time to fully digest. Compare that with a half cup of apple juice (I don't know how many apples it takes to make a half cup of juice, but I'm sure it's more than one). The apple juice is not going to make your stomach feel full, but the two cups of apple will.

The food industry likes us to eat refined/processed foods because we will buy and eat more of them at one time. Then, when they disappear quickly through digestion and our stomach feels empty, we will buy and eat more again. Good for the food industry; not good for us.

Protein and fat. Bulk will fill the volume of your stomach, but by itself cannot always keep you full because your body needs more than bulk. Many current diet recommendations have mistakenly assumed that bulk can take the place of protein and fat. They suggest that a large quantity of something like raw veggies or a cooked vegetable (with a low- or non-fat dressing) or even water will stave off your hunger if you eat/drink enough of it. But they totally miss that bulk isn't the only contributor to satisfaction. Sometimes your body needs something different.

The standard edict is that to be healthy you need to stick to low-fat foods. But processed low-fat foods have additives and sweeteners to make them palatable. They stimulate your hunger rather than satisfy it. And naturally low-fat foods like vegetables taste better with the addition of some fat. That's why so-called healthy foods get such a bad reputation. Quality foods can be combined so that you get a satisfying proportion of carbohydrates, protein, and fat that will keep you satisfied for hours.

To get a little more specific:
- 100 calories of real, unadulterated cheesecake (even though this is a small quantity) will satisfy me longer than 100 calories of artificially sweetened non-fat yogurt.

- One hundred calories of real cheese (about one ounce) will last me longer than two hundred calories of reduced-fat cheese.
- A salad with a good olive-oil-and-vinegar dressing will last longer than a salad with fat-free, sugar-laden dressing.
- I would rather have one tablespoon of real sour cream than a quarter cup of the fat-free variety.

I'm happier and my body is happier too.

The satisfaction factor is a real problem. When you're hungry you'll obsess about food and will eat too much. When you're truly satisfied you won't obsess about food, and you'll eat less. *Quantity cannot trump quality*. Real, whole foods are deeply satisfying and they don't leave you in a constant state of craving.

HOW TO IDENTIFY WHOLE FOODS

Defining quality foods

The following is the best definition of healthy food I've found; it's a report by the Washington statewide Access to Healthy Foods Coalition (which was disbanded in 2013). It's unfortunately, no longer available online, but here's the text:

> *A healthy food is a plant or animal product that provides essential nutrients and energy to sustain growth, health, and life while satiating hunger.*
>
> *Healthy foods are usually fresh or minimally processed foods, naturally dense in nutrients, that when eaten in moderation and in combination with other foods, sustain growth, repair and maintain vital processes, promote longevity, reduce disease, and strengthen and maintain the body and its functions.*
>
> *Healthy foods do not contain ingredients that contribute to disease or impede recovery when consumed at normal levels.*

I fully agree with this definition. However, I choose to use the term *quality* foods rather than *healthy* foods. The general use of the term *healthy* has been rendered meaningless by government policy, food-industry marketing, so-called health foods, the mass media, and probably by other sources as well. By now, consumers are so jaded about what healthy food is, they associate the term with something that lacks taste and satisfaction. What I hear in casual conversation and see reflected in the media is, "If it tastes good, it can't possibly be good for you" or phrased in the reverse, "If it's good for you, it can't possibly taste good." An acquaintance once commented,

"When I hear someone talk about healthy food, my eyes glaze over." The message consumers have absorbed is that pleasure and health are mutually exclusive.

And this is unfortunate, as it sets up a strong psychological conflict: if we eat the food we think is healthy we feel we've done the right thing but we're unsatisfied and we miss our unhealthy food; if we eat the food we love we're satisfied but we feel guilty.

Winning the Battle of Quality will show you that this line of thinking is wrong.

What makes a food a quality food?

You can't identify a quality food solely by the following product-label statistics per serving because these stats don't give you the right kind of information.

The criteria I use to identify a quality food

- Closeness to its original source (measured as steps in processing)
- How it was processed
- What it does *not* contain
- Freshness

Not all foods will pass or fail all the tests, and sometimes you have to decide where to draw the line. However, when you start to apply those tests you'll quickly see that all real, whole foods will pass and heavily processed foods will fail.

Closeness to its original source

I don't mean closeness geographically. I am referring to the number of processing steps between the original and the final product. For instance, the steps between an apple on a tree and an apple in the store might be washing with water and spraying with an edible wax, so an apple is very close to its original source. A made-from-scratch cake is somewhat close to its source if it's made with basic ingredients, such as unbleached flour, milk, butter, eggs, and sugar. On the other hand, a cake made from a boxed mix is not close to its original source because every ingredient in it has been subjected to multiple processes: the flour is highly refined; the milk and eggs are powdered; it likely has multiple sources of sweeteners, additives, and preservatives; and so on.

How it's processed

Processing can be enhancing, neutral, or destructive. Natural fermentation *enhances* products like cheese, yogurt, and soy. Freezing is *neutral*: it doesn't change the basic nutrition. *Destructive* refers to how much refinement has been done to the original and what additives have been used to get to the end product. With a whole-grain hot cereal such as steel-cut oats, the oats have simply been pressed and sliced—a minimally destructive process. For most children's cereals, the original primary ingredient (wheat, rice, corn, etc.) is completely taken apart and reassembled in some kid-friendly shape with lots of artificial flavors and sugar—a highly destructive process.

Destructive is what you should try to avoid.

What it does NOT contain

By this I mean that the simpler the list of ingredients, the better. Foods do not need a long list of additives and preservatives to make them taste good. And while it might be creative to give products various flavorings that don't naturally occur in a food, these low-quality food products usually rely on an artificial means of adding those flavors. Plain potato chips consist of potatoes, oil, and salt—simple, and except for a little too much salt, tasty. But when you get into barbecue, ranch, and other enhanced flavors suddenly the list of ingredients expands to include a host of unidentifiable additives. Same with natural vs. flavored nuts. Quality foods do not contain these enhancers.

One thing to be aware of is that some chemical-sounding additives are actually forms of vitamins you don't have to avoid, so it's a good idea to become familiar with those. *Tocopherol*, for instance, is a form of vitamin E and it's used to stabilize oils and other products that have had their natural vitamin E removed. *Thiamine* is the chemical name for Vitamin B1. *Nicotinic acid,* which sounds terrible, is just the chemical term for Niacin (Vitamin B3).

Most additives and preservatives in food have been approved by the Food and Drug Administration (FDA) and as such, are supposed to be safe. But not everyone agrees with FDA approvals, and it can be very complicated to follow the studies to try to figure it out for yourself. A few of the more common ones are monosodium glutamate (MSG), high-fructose corn syrup, azodicarbonamide (ADA), carrageenan, guar gum, xanthan gum, potassium bromate, mono-and di-glycerides, and sodium stearoyl lactate. If you really want a full list and the nitty-gritty details, get a copy of *A Consumer's Dictionary of Food Additives, 7th Edition,* by Ruth Winter.

On the other hand, you can keep it simple: just avoid as many additives and preservatives as you can because they're there to make up for deficiencies created by processing. Whole foods don't need to be doctored.

Freshness

I especially want to clarify what I mean by freshness because the term *fresh* has been hijacked for marketing hype. The real meaning of a fresh food is that both the end product and the ingredients have been *recently made* or recently harvested. There is also an implication that it doesn't contain additives or preservatives because presumably, if it's really fresh it doesn't need any.

The new meaning of fresh for marketing purposes is limited to *recently made*. For example, supermarket bakeries and some chain stores may offer fresh bread, but it's only freshly *baked*—the dough may be heavily processed or have been trucked in from some central location where it's made with plenty of additives and preservatives and stored for weeks or months. For another example, while lunchmeat can be freshly *sliced*, most of it contains a heavy dose of additives and preservatives; it's not fresh in the true sense.

The freshness test should also apply to foods grown in foreign countries and shipped here over thousands of miles. We've become used to having every kind of fruit and vegetable at any time of the year. But only those grown relatively locally in their usual season are really fresh. That doesn't mean that the shipped ones have no value, they're just less fresh and you can tell that from the lack of taste. One exception is vegetables and fruits that have been flash-frozen soon after harvest so they retain most of their original nutritional elements.

The bottom line is that if there are no additives or preservatives involved, it's pretty easy to tell if a food is fresh or not. If it isn't fresh it shows signs of deterioration: discoloration, mold, odor, or limp texture. You can also tell by how fast it goes bad after you buy it and take it home. If a product contains preservatives, it isn't fresh.

Bread as an example

Closeness to its original source. Bread made from 100 percent whole wheat is close to its original source because the wheat still contains all its edible parts. Bread made from refined white flour is not close because this wheat has been stripped of its natural nutrition.

How it was processed. Bread dough has to be kneaded, but large bread manufacturers process both white and wheat bread with dough conditioners to make kneading large quantities easier for their machines. Most manufacturers add a variety of additives and preservatives as well. A quality bread is made without the conditioners, additives, and preservatives.

What it does not contain. Watch out for additives such as potassium bromate, mono-and di-glycerides, sodium stearoyl lactate, partially hydrogenated oils, calcium propionate, dextrose, L-cysteine, Azodicarbonamide, high-fructose corn syrup, and others.

The simplest bread consists of flour, water, salt, and yeast and optionally a tiny bit of sugar or honey. Other common natural ingredients are milk, butter or vegetable oil, and eggs. True artisan (usually meaning mostly hand-made) breads limit themselves to these basic ingredients with other natural foods for various flavors: rosemary, olive, garlic, and so on. Regardless of the type of flour (white, whole wheat, rye, etc.) you can identify a quality bread by the absence of non-bread-related ingredients.

Freshness. A bread is only truly fresh if it has no additives or preservatives and it has been made within the last day or two, at most. The only way you can know for sure if the bread is truly fresh is by reading the label (date and ingredients) or asking for a list of ingredients from the bakery.

The bottom line: Quality foods = real, whole foods

When identifying quality foods it's much easier to summarize what *is* than what is not. Real food means it occurs naturally and is not manufactured by the food industry as a value-added product. Whole food means it contains most of the nutrients it had when it was harvested.

There are too many real foods to list specifically, but broadly speaking, here are the more common whole foods:

- Vegetables—fresh, frozen (without sauces), canned with no additives other than salt, a little sugar, and herb flavorings
- Dried beans
- Fruits (fresh, frozen without added sugar)
- Whole grains (some of these are revived ancient grains)
- Baked goods made from natural ingredients such as flour (any variety but without additives), butter, oil, eggs, milk or cream, sugar, and natural flavorings
- Proteins (fish, beef, chicken, lamb, pork, eggs, wild game—preferably raised without hormones and antibiotics and minimally processed, and *not* the prepackaged versions like fish sticks or chicken nuggets)
- Fats (vegetable oils, butter, nut oils, minimally processed—look for "cold pressed" on the label)

- Dairy products (whole)
- Nuts (minimally processed and not artificially flavored)
- Beverages (unsweetened or lightly naturally sweetened, wine, beer, other alcohol, etc.)
- Fresh and dried spices (without additives)
- Snack foods with only additives such as a little salt, sugar and/or herb flavorings
- Sugars (such as honey, cane, molasses)

A word about sugars. Sugars add variety to our food flavors, and as long as they're consumed in small quantities (even refined sugar) they're not likely to cause health problems. There is no reason to become fanatical about it. For example, it isn't unusual to find Thai recipes that call for palm sugar, and the Thai diet is considered healthy. Apply the 80/20 rule: if 80 percent of what you eat is quality, the other 20 percent isn't going to kill you. Eating should be enjoyable and there's nothing wrong with an occasional use of some variety of sugar.

There is a lot of buzz about the sweetener Stevia. I didn't include this in my list because while this is a somewhat natural product, it's intensely sweet and I think the problem with something like that is it perpetuates the craving for sweet foods.

You can get nitpicky about it, but you don't need to. While it's mostly true that vegetables and fruits from a farmers' market are higher in quality than those at a supermarket, organic is better than non-organic, meat from a local farm is better than factory-farmed meat, and wild fish is better than farmed fish, wherever you find foods in the real/whole category will be good enough; the difference is not that great. No need to go crazy. The most important distinction to make is between whole foods and processed foods.

HOW TO IDENTIFY PROCESSED FOODS

Now that you have the identifiers for quality foods, it's easy to categorize processed foods: they fall under "everything else." The reason for identifying processed foods is that they're the ones you need to replace. Notice, I did *not* say *avoid*. *Resetting Normal* does not require you to avoid foods, but to find whole foods that you like just as well or better than their processed counterparts and eat them instead. *Over time,* you *replace* the bad with the good. You don't *pull* them out leaving a void, you *push* them out with something better and tastier.

Figuring out what to replace should be easy now: any food that is not mostly whole should be replaced or at least reduced. However, not all food processing is bad. Almost every food we eat is processed in some way, and many are perfectly healthy. But at some point, processing crosses the line into unhealthy, and that is what I will try to quantify here.

Truly unprocessed foods

Strictly speaking, the only legitimately unprocessed foods are those that come directly from nature. That would only include raw vegetables, fruits and nuts, untreated; raw meat and fat from animals, fish, reptiles, or bugs that consumed only their natural diets, not treated with hormones or antibiotics; and unpasteurized dairy products. One could even argue that only meat from wild animals rather than domesticated ones like cattle or chickens would qualify, but that's a little extreme.

But people have been processing foods naturally for thousands of years. The methods they invented made foods taste better, easier to digest, and safer; prevented spoilage; and in some cases even added nutritional value. How do you have enough to eat through the winter months or through a drought if you can't preserve food in some way? So first, a quick look at processed foods that are *acceptable* and likely to be available in the modern world.

Processing methods that get the stamp of approval

Most of these have been used for centuries and when done naturally, add value and render foods more palatable and digestible. They include:

- Cooking
- Drying
- Curing (usually with salt)
- Smoking
- Freezing
- Preserving with sugar
- Fermenting (cheese, soy, beer, etc.)
- Pickling
- Pressing (to extract oils)
- Canning
- Treating with lye (masa, olives)

How modern processing is bad for us

The basic goal of capitalism is to continually make more money. In the agriculture/food industry, this means *optimization*. I've got nothing against reasonable efficiency, but it has gone too far. Here are the negative effects of this optimization:

- Shipping globally takes time during which nutritive elements deteriorate.
- Monoculture reduces variety.
- Massive centralized processing includes adding hormones and antibiotics to animal feed, passing them on to us.
- We consume chemicals that are added to speed up processing and we lose the value of longer fermentation.
- We consume extra salt and sugar added to increase product weight.
- We consume artificial flavor enhancers and preservatives added to increase shelf life.
- We consume extremely refined faux foods with little or no nutritional value.
- We consume more than we need because designer foods go down so fast our internal appetite controls don't work .

Many would say that this optimization allows more people to have more food. Yes, that's true. With the rapid increase in world population, so many more people living in cities, and fewer people farming the land, there are logistical challenges to providing *fresh* food for everyone[16]. Agribusiness and the food industry have certainly met those challenges. But the problem of not having enough food has morphed into something else: we have quantity, but we've sacrificed quality. We can eat and eat to fill our stomachs, but our body inside is still hungry because it never gets what it really needs.

The underlying problem is that we've come to think of today's processed foods as normal and we accept chemical ingredients without question. At work I saw a box of cupcakes on the kitchen counter that someone had left with the good intention of sharing something sweet with co-workers. I couldn't help myself; I had to read the label. And the ingredients were so far from real I had to copy them down for this book. It's a glaring example of one common food item that contains more non-food ingredients than real food.

First, for a basis of comparison, here are the ingredients for simple real vanilla or chocolate cupcakes with icing:

Real cupcakes: Enriched white flour (not bleached), sugar, cocoa, baking powder or baking soda, eggs, milk, butter or vegetable oil, vanilla (not artificial vanillin)

Real icing: Butter, confectioner's sugar, vanilla

Real toppings: Nuts, chocolate chips, coconut, dried fruit

Now, below is the list of ingredients from the boxed cupcakes from the supermarket. I have separated the list into *real* and *artificial ingredients*. And as you can see, the artificial ones outnumber the real ones.

Real ingredients: Sugar, cocoa, dried egg whites, nonfat dry milk, dried egg yolks, leavening, salt

Artificial, refined ingredients: Bleached enriched wheat flour, Partially hydrogenated vegetable oil (soybean/cottonseed oil, propylene glycol monoester, mono & diglycerides), modified food starch, dextrose, natural and artificial flavor, Polysorbate 60, Tetrasodium pyrophosphate, corn syrup solids, gum Arabic, Sodium propionate (preservative), calcium acetate, guar gum, xanthan gum, potassium sorbate (preservative), Red 40 (color)

Real frosting ingredients: Butter, sugar, water, dried egg whites, cream of tartar, salt, cocoa powder

Artificial, refined frosting ingredients: Corn syrup, Sorbitol, Microcrystalline cellulose, sodium stearoyl lactylate, glucomodeltalactone, sodium alginate, vegetable oils (soy and palm), soy lecithin (emulsifier), corn starch, vanillin (artificial vanilla flavor), tocopherol (antioxidant)

Real ingredients included in "Toppings may contain": Corn starch, confectioner's glaze, rice

Artificial ingredients included in "Toppings may contain": Carnauba wax, artificial color (FD&C Red 40, FD&C Yellow #6, FD&C Blue #2, FD&C Yellow #5, FD&C Red #2, FD&C Blue #1, Red 40 Lake, Yellow 6 Lake, Blue 1 Lake, Yellow 5 Lake, Green 3), partially hydrogenated vegetable oil (cottonseed, soybean), dextrin, soy lecithin (emulsifier)

There are absolutely no redeeming qualities about these cupcakes, and this is not an extreme example. I can guarantee you there are many, many products just like this on the market and people eat them every day, thinking they're actually food.

A SUMMARY OF WHAT TO REPLACE

Since the majority of foods in the supermarket are highly processed and new ones are being invented all the time, it would be impossible to list them all here and have that list up to date. You can apply the general guidelines for identifying processed foods (from the earlier section). But here are a few categories to look for:

- Boxed mixes

- Frozen food entrees (except for the newer, more natural ones)
- White bread
- Artificially prepared alternatives to bacon and sausage
- Any protein foods labeled "nuggets"
- Seasoning packets with multiple flavor enhancers and preservatives, such as MSG
- Fat-free salad dressings
- Artificially flavored snack foods
- Sodas—including low-cal, sugar-free, diet, etc.
- Food products with a lot of added sugars
- Sugared cereals
- Artificial foods like whipped toppings

What if you're vegetarian or vegan?

Lots of processed products on the market are aimed at you. And as the food industry increasingly co-opts the term "vegan," expect an increase in unhealthy vegan foods. The vegetarian or vegan label gives them the aura of healthy, but many of them are high in flavor enhancers, sugars, additives and preservatives. You need to be vigilant about reading ingredient labels to weed them out. There are plenty of real, quality foods available to you, however, and if you stick with those you're on the right track. Just watch out for some soy products, highly flavored and sweetened almond and rice milks, highly sweetened desserts, and so on.

There's no need to be fanatical

It's virtually impossible to replace all processed foods. But while one single product may have only a small amount, if you eat a lot of those products the junk adds up, and that's what you should try to prevent. There's still a place for some processed products, and there's no need to panic unless you have a specific allergic reaction to a particular additive or preservative. For example, I avoid MSG (monosodium glutamate) because it's a concentrated flavor enhancer that messes with how the brain perceives taste, and I'd just as soon not consume it. It has many names, including yeast extract, so it's sometimes hard to identify. For a list of these names, see Alternate Names for Monosodium Glutamate in *Appendix C*. It's also in just about every processed food there is (in one of its many forms). But if I ate some food with yeast extract in it I wouldn't run around screaming "OMG! OMG! I just swallowed some yeast extract!" I just generally avoid it when possible.

Why avoiding processed foods is a challenge

There are two reasons it's difficult to avoid processed foods:
1) They're everywhere—in some areas processed food is the only kind that local stores carry.
2) We are so used to them we think of them as the normal thing to eat.

The food industry claims all their additives have been sanctioned by the FDA and they cite multiple studies that support these claims. This position allows them to keep flooding the market with these products. But there are three glaring omissions of the supporting studies:
1) None of them are long term enough to assess the cumulative effect of consuming the additives and preservatives regularly over a lifetime.
2) They don't account for the effect of the absent nutrients.
3) There is the question of industry influence in FDA decisions.

We've come to accept the notion that if the food wasn't good for us, it wouldn't be in the store. Surely the FDA wouldn't have approved it otherwise. Right ... but because the changeover from whole foods to processed ones occurred gradually and with our welcome (convenience over substance), we've lost sight of how to tell the difference.

Still, we can fight back by educating ourselves about how to improve the quality of our foods.

ANSWERS TO POTENTIAL QUESTIONS

If I stick to whole foods, will I still have plenty of tasty choices?

Now that I've defined what I mean by quality foods in a general way and given the reasons I think they're best, it's time to get specific. What makes it worth the time and trouble to replace processed foods with quality foods? Does it limit your choices? Does it really taste good? Do you have to replace all processed foods?

The variety of whole foods available to most of us today is exceptional. While chicken, steaks, and other meats, and a wide variety of vegetables and fruits are most reasonably priced in their raw form, the food industry has seen the demand for whole foods rise steadily over the past twenty years and has stepped in with freshly prepared and frozen options for convenience. Practically every supermarket offers meats cut to size for any preparation, bagged vegetable mixes and salads, and ready-to-eat fruit. And many of these items only require a few minutes in a microwave. We just need to know how to cut through the marketing hype, how to identify the good stuff, and how to prepare it quickly.

How does this apply to various dietary food patterns?

Whether you consider yourself an omnivore, a vegetarian, or a vegan, you can be healthy or unhealthy with any one of these dietary patterns, depending on which foods you choose. If you're comfortable being an omnivore, there's no reason to change that. If you're comfortable as a vegetarian or vegan, that's fine too. It's much more important that the foods you select are mostly whole. To reset normal you have to choose the appropriate *quality* foods for your particular dietary pattern. There are real, whole foods available in each category and there are refined, processed, junky foods available in each category.

What about organic vs. regular?

If organic choices are available and not cost-prohibitive, use them. If not, don't worry about it; there is plenty of nutrition in regular real foods and if nothing else, our industrialized farm system makes them readily available at a reasonable price. You'll get the most benefit from choosing real foods (organic or not) over processed foods. In a perfect world, it would be easy and affordable to buy organic, farm-raised foods and avoid the hidden junk. But it isn't always, and we have to work with the world we have.

What about farm-raised meats?

Aside from the moral reasons for humane treatment of factory-farmed animals, meat from grass-fed animals is superior to their industrialized equivalents. However, the same thing applies here as for organic vs. regular: if it's not available and/or too expensive, you'll still be better off choosing the industrial-sourced meats over processed foods.

What about local vs. long-distance?

Some foods travel better than others. Fresh foods like vegetables and fruits don't—they quickly lose their nutrients, and breeding them for travel destroys their texture, taste, and nutritional content. Foods that travel well include: coffee beans, cocoa beans, dried beans, potatoes, carrots (vegetables that don't bruise easily and store well), bananas, pineapple, meat, frozen fruits and vegetables, grains like wheat, and rice. Fish is a toss-up. It's best very fresh but isn't available everywhere locally, so it travels to some of us frozen.

It's best if you can get most of your foods locally, but with a growing population, that may not be possible. I see nothing wrong with importing foods unique to certain geographic areas (bananas, coffee, pineapple, cocoa beans, etc.). These are foods we can all enjoy and there's no reason why the people of these areas should not benefit from selling their unique produce, as long as we pay them a fair price.

Is more real food always better?

As with anything, more is not always better. I'm always skeptical of trendy diet ideas like juicing when they're based on the idea that if you drink the juice of ten carrots you'll get ten times the nutrition. First of all, when you juice a carrot (and other fruits and vegetables), you lose much of the fiber. Second, what makes anyone think we need ten times the nutritional elements of one carrot at one time? Vitamins and minerals are used in the context of our metabolism. Just because we need x grams of a vitamin to be healthy doesn't mean ten times that is even healthier.

Frequently we see hype about potential silver bullets: foods that are supposed to be so special, if we eat enough of them that will guarantee our health. Whether it's acai berries, green coffee beans, green tea, goji berries, vitamin C, wheatgrass, probiotics, ginseng, ginkgo biloba, or some other food, vitamin or mineral, *there is no single nutritional element that will give you a long, healthy life.* Some of them may be a part of a healthy diet, but don't waste your money counting on only one thing; it's not a good strategy in the stock market and not good in your diet. Eating real from a wide variety of foods is your best insurance plan.

Sometimes more is not better, it's toxic.

What about "smoothies"?

A *smoothie* is a drink made in a blender. Ingredients vary, but usually include fat-free plain or flavored yogurt, soy milk, soft tofu, or kefir as a base. Additional ingredients include fruit, fruit juice, seeds, nuts, protein powder, honey, sugar, artificial sweeteners, and even vegetables like spinach or kale. Sounds healthy, right? The problem is that the quality of these drinks can vary widely, depending on what goes into them. A smoothie made from whole foods like whole yogurt, fruit, nuts, and vegetables can be refreshing once in a while. But I have the following objections:

- Flavored, fat-free yogurt is a processed food with additives.
- Protein powder is a processed food.
- Added natural sweeteners make these concoctions high in sugar (usually more than sixteen grams and sometimes as much as fifty grams).
- Artificial sweeteners are not healthy additives.

One other thing to consider. As I've noted, *the package matters*, and in the case of a smoothie made entirely from whole-food ingredients, the package is still there—sort of. However, the digestive process, including appestat signaling, starts in your mouth when you chew your food. When you drink a smoothie, no chewing is required, so it bypasses the early start of digestion and appetite signaling. In addition, because the blending processes the food so finely, your stomach will have less work to do to break it down and you need much less time to consume it, shortening the pleasure of eating it. The result is that digestion time is shorter and you won't be satisfied for as long as you would if you ate all the ingredients separately, unblended.

My conclusion about smoothies is that when they're made with whole ingredients and no added sugar, they won't hurt now and then. When you're in a bind for a quick lunch or a seriously needed snack, they can be a reasonable occasional choice. But using them regularly as meal replacements is not the best idea.

What about cooking methods?

You don't have to limit yourself to steamed vegetables and broiled meats. Frying is not the best preparation because heating some oils to a high temperature causes them to break down into trans fats. However, if you choose your oil correctly, some frying is not going to harm you. Although the experts won't tell you this, the best oils to fry with are those that are completely saturated (like lard) because a saturated fat is stable and doesn't disintegrate at high temperatures like many vegetable oils. The standard peanut oil and corn oil don't have much nutritional value because they've been refined and processed to tolerate high temperatures, but at least they're stable. Stir-frying and sautéing can be done with just about any fat if the pan temperature isn't too high.

Even if you don't like cooking, there are methods that make preparation of whole foods practically painless. When I was working full-time, my work plus commute time took twelve hours and frequently I arrived home at six-thirty needing to get dinner on the table by six-forty-five or seven. Believe it or not, with a little planning, it's possible to do this with whole foods. See the companion website at ***resettingnormal.com*** for a how-to.

What about ready-made food products?

No one has the time these days to make everything from the basic ingredients; we're all going to buy some things ready-made. This is where label reading comes in. When buying ready-made products, look for those made with only (or almost only) whole foods. But try to see through the healthy hype. For example, plain potato chips have a bad rap because the potatoes are fried in oil, so manufacturers started producing a baked variety. But look at the label. I haven't seen one yet for baked chips that doesn't include highly refined starches, sugar, and other additives.

You're better off with plain, regular potato chips made with sunflower, corn or canola oil. The ingredients should be simple: potatoes, oil, and salt. Just don't eat the whole bag.

Only a decade ago it was almost impossible to find ready-made food products without additives and preservatives, but enough people have become concerned with what's in their food that the food industry has responded by providing more natural choices.

CONTROVERSIES

Many experts discourage us from consuming some whole foods like whole milk, butter, red meat, and so on. I'd like to supply my reasons for claiming these foods have a place in a healthy, quality diet. The underlying principle is that whole foods help you reset normal. They not only provide the nutrition and the satisfaction that let your internal appestat take control, but they make eating pleasurable.

If you have an allergy or genuine intolerance for a particular whole food or an aversion based on ethical reasons, fine. But don't translate that into avoiding all whole foods that have a bad rap from many experts. Eating should not be about deprivation. It should not be reduced to a battle of will power. Select whole foods you can enjoy.

Low-fat craziness

Real foods are powerhouses of nutrition, but if you're not allowed to prepare them so that they taste good, you're not going to eat them. Salad is great for you but not very satisfying with fake nonfat dressing or just lemon juice. And fat-free dressings are so full of sweeteners they just make you hungrier. While an olive-oil-based dressing would be ideal, even if you only like a mayonnaise-based dressing, use it—you'll still get the benefits that come with the salad. I hear experts claim that adding this kind of dressing completely nullifies the benefit of the salad, but that's crazy. You're still going to get the vitamins and minerals from it; the dressing isn't going to take those away. A better approach is to use the dressing but use it sparingly.

For another example, consider broccoli—a whole, quality food by itself. But you don't have to eat it plain. Maybe you like broccoli but only with butter or cheese sauce. Are you better off skipping it altogether to avoid eating the butter or sauce? Should you force yourself to eat it plain? Or should you eat it the way you like it? Broccoli contains a boatload of nutrition and considerable fiber so if the only way you'll eat it is with the butter or sauce, do it. Forcing yourself to eat it plain will just cause you to compensate with something else later or will make you learn to dislike it altogether.

Low-fat craziness also leads to absurdities. When the food industry mixes up experts' low-fat, low-calorie health messages with its own marketing agendas, we are required to navigate the resulting ridiculousness.
Examples:

- A coffee shop that does not serve whole-milk lattes (because whole milk has a bad reputation of saturated fat), yet they do serve gigantic eight-inch, trans-fat-laden, sugar-filled cinnamon rolls. It's ok to have all that stuff in the pastry but not the four grams of saturated fat in a latte?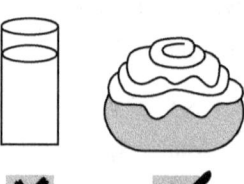
- "Thinny chips" (low-calorie, low-fat) served at a work lunch next to monster four-inch chocolate chip cookies for dessert. Please tell me why it's not ok to have regular potato chips, but it is ok to have the huge cookies.
- Diet soda (no-calorie) making people feel better about consuming meals with 2,000 or more calories. Like the lack of calories in the soda is going to make a difference?
- Most yogurts on the market are either low-fat or non-fat. Yet these versions are so unpalatable plain, the manufacturers have to fill them with sugar (or artificial sweetener), additives, and flavorings to make them acceptable to American taste. These concoctions cannot possibly be healthier then plain, full-fat yogurt.

When you grasp an understanding of these absurdities, you can at least try not to get sucked in by them, and you can point them out to others (in a humorous way).

Foods with saturated fat

Most of the whole-foods experts warn us away from are foods that contain saturated fat. This includes dairy products, red meat, bacon, and other similar foods. I still say it comes down to quantity; there's nothing wrong with these foods in reasonable quantities. Besides, some new studies indicate that saturated fat might not be the dietary evil it was previously thought to be.

If you enjoy these foods but try to refrain from eating any, you'll just end up binging on them at some point. For example, one company breakfast provided an awesome feast, including some excellent alder-smoked bacon. I watched with amusement as people took the paper cups intended for juice and filled them with bacon. What I heard were comments like, "I know I'm not supposed to eat this but it's here, and it's so good I might as well fill up while I have a chance."

If you worry about your saturated-fat consumption, you can always limit the quantities and still allow yourself to feed your body what it needs, eating whatever whole foods you want while keeping some types of nutrients in check. It will give you the greatest satisfaction and put a stop to your cravings, which means you'll eat less food overall.

Soy: yes or no?

I'm ambivalent about soy products even though they've been crowned with the health aura. From a personal standpoint, I don't tolerate them well due to the high level of phytoestrogens, and I avoid anything that contains soy protein isolates. Naturally fermented soy products are deemed quite healthy, but can be hard to find and even harder to tell if they're naturally fermented or not. Whole soy beans are natural, but all other soy products are highly processed with many additives, and that makes them suspect in my view.

Still, many vegetarians and vegans depend on soy products for their primary source of protein and seem to do fine with them. I recommend that if you consume a lot of soy, even if you stick with whole soy beans, you watch for any symptoms that seem to be abnormal. Otherwise, it's open for you to determine if you want or need to include them in your diet.

Exceptions to the whole-foods rule

While I believe whole foods are best, some cultures have managed to stay quite healthy even though some of their staple foods are not whole according to my definition. The most obvious of these foods is white rice, used as a staple in Asian cultures. Also, the French have a history of making excellent white breads and pastries, and as long as they maintain their traditional French diet, they manage to stay quite healthy. These cultures do, however, balance their diets by consuming such foods in reasonable quantities, making up the rest of their diet with whole foods and maintaining an active lifestyle.

You can't go wrong with real

Day after day we're assaulted with reports of studies about the latest food we shouldn't eat. If we aligned our diets with those studies, there would be about ten foods left. We'd have to conclude that everything else causes cancer, heart disease, and diabetes. So forget the studies.

The basic guideline for what to eat to win the Battle of Quality is that you can choose any combination of real, whole, quality foods, every one of which has nutritional value. Start out with no restrictions; just get used to eating and enjoying whole foods. Enjoy the new tastes and savor the textures of whole, natural foods without worrying about *how much* you're eating. Don't go hungry. But learn these new flavors and find the ones you really like.

Once you have switched most of your diet to real, whole foods you can tweak it in any direction you want. If you want to move to a lower-fat diet, you'll be able to do that. If you want to eat less red meat, you'll be able to do that. Your own built-in appestat will take over and guide you as to the type and quantity of food you need at any given time. No outside expert or computer program can do that for you.

NOTES

BEAT THE MARKETING MACHINE

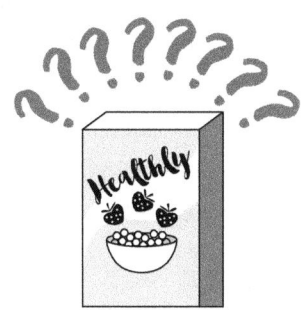

The Marketing Machine uses what I call buzzwords and bear traps to get you to buy their products. The buzzwords are designed to make you think a product is healthy—this is the bait. If you take the bait you're likely to fall into the bear traps, which are scenarios that play on your beliefs about what is healthy and what fits your lifestyle and budget. For example, if a product is labeled "low-fat" and you believe a low-fat diet is healthy, you're likely to buy it without considering any of the negative aspects of the product.

Action #1: Learn the marketing buzzwords

Now that you know how to identify whole foods vs. processed foods, it's time to build your defenses against misleading marketing practices that make consumers think processed food is a better choice than the real, whole-food equivalent. To reset normal, you'll need be aware of all the marketing traps so you're not tricked. You should welcome this challenge because *aren't you really, really tired of being manipulated and deceived?* I surely am. The food industry takes the latest health advice and spins it in ways to make their products appear healthy, whether they are or not.

The Merriam-Webster Dictionary defines *buzzword* as an important-sounding, usually technical word or phrase, often of little meaning, used chiefly to impress laypersons. Remember, the food industry's goal is to sell us stuff, preferably a lot of stuff, and it has learned to dazzle us with buzzwords that confer an aura of health to bear-trap us into becoming loyal customers. One of the things you'll need to do reset normal is to commercial-proof yourself against this marketing strategy, so it's really important to understand which terms have a legitimate meaning and which do not.

This list morphs all the time in response to target markets that experts inadvertently create with their recommendations. The food industry co-opts that latest "health-speak" to attract customers. Below is a table showing a small sample of these target markets and the buzzwords associated with them. Look for new ones on the companion website.

While a given buzzword might be *partially* appropriate for a product, the manufacturer's goal is to trap you into buying it regardless. Usually (but not always) this means diverting your attention from other ingredients in the product that aren't healthful. For example, a product might be labeled organic but contain large amounts of sugar and/or salt. It could be labeled high-protein but contain a long list of additives. It could be labeled fat-busting—but what does that even mean? So the difficulty is distinguishing which products are labeled truthfully and which are not. And the only way you can do that is to *ignore the product's buzzword and read the complete ingredients label.*

Target Market	Buzzwords
Fear of fat	Low-fat, fat-free, 0 trans fat, Omega 3, Omega 6
Fear of carbs	0 grams of carbs, low-carb, sugar-free, no added sugar
Looking for special health benefits	Antioxidants, powerful antioxidants, soy, cholesterol-free, lycopene, heart healthy, vegan, smart, superfood, skinny foods, vitamin-rich, protein-packed, real (as in "real" protein)
Looking for wholesomeness and purity	Organic, natural, all natural, 100 percent natural, whole grain, multi-grain, fresh, made fresh, fresh taste, farmer's, wholesome, home, homestyle, artisanal (originally "handcrafted," now co-opted by large companies), honest
Looking for potential metabolic benefits	High-protein, low-glycemic, gluten-free, high-fiber, pro-biotic
Hoping for weight loss	Low-calorie, flat-belly foods, fat-busting, fat-burner
Confident in the approval of science	Scientifically formulated, clinically proven

It's important to point out that some of the products using buzzwords actually are quality foods. But many are not. Same advice: don't be fooled by the name—read the label details. The product might be as advertised, but you won't know for sure unless you check what's in it. Do your homework and you won't fall into the product-label trap.

Here are some examples of products with buzzwords in their names that imply health:

- Campbell's *Healthy Request* soups
- Oscar Mayer *DeliFresh* lunchmeats
- Hormel *Natural Choice* lunchmeats
- *Nature Valley* granola bars
- Kashi *Organic Promise* cereals
- Kroger *Simple Truth* product line
- Any product names that include thin, skinny, smart, lean, honest, natural,

artisan, fresh, or fruit (for products aimed at kids) leverage buzzwords with a healthy aura.

Your Action here is just to become familiar with the common buzzwords; see if you can identify them in advertising and on product packaging.

Action #2: Practice identifying the buzzwords

Don't take the buzzword bait. When you hear or see one of these buzzwords, raise your warning antenna—*beep, beep, beep*! Avoid the Jedi mind trick to draw your attention away from the negative and possibly more important aspects of the product. You should immediately stop, engage your brain, read the whole label, and ask yourself questions. How much sugar does each serving contain? Does it contain artificial sweeteners? What additives and preservatives are included? Does it contain partially hydrogenated fats? What fillers (gums, texture enhancers)?

Believe it or not, there are plenty of truly natural food products on the market that taste great and don't have all the additive junk. If we all bought those and didn't buy products based on the buzzwords, the food industry would change. Marketers use health buzzwords because they work: consumers spend more of their hard-earned cash for these products, and the food industry profits.

Choose ten common products in your food supply. Write down the marketing buzzwords on each package, if any. Then ask yourself these questions:

- Who do you think is the company's target market?
- What is it about those words that make you feel like the product is healthy and safe?
- Compare the buzzwords with the list of ingredients. Does the buzzword distract you from the bad ingredients in the product?
- Do you really benefit from this product, or is the company merely trying to persuade you to buy it because it generates more profit for them?

Action #3: Learn to recognize the bear traps

The bear traps are designed with the understanding that most of us want to buy products that are healthy, convenient, effective, and inexpensive. Learning to recognize these traps may require you to question some of your underlying assumptions about these characteristics.

The low-/non-fat trap

When you see a label that claims to be low- or non-fat, read what else is in it. The vast majority of processed products labeled low- or non-fat contain additives that give them a fat-like texture, and depending on the nature of the product, a variety of sweeteners, extra salt, and probably some form of MSG. Seriously, if low- and non-fat products worked to help people lose weight and be healthy, there would be no obesity or chronic health problems today. If you're convinced of the healthfulness of a low-fat eating pattern, you can craft one using real, whole foods without spending money on the faux junk.

The low-calorie trap

Basing your food choices solely on calories is a bad idea. Food value is much more important than the number of calories. Probably the worst low-calorie trap arrived with the invention of diet soda. The holy grail of the food industry is selling you something that makes you think you can consume it in unlimited quantities (zero calories, zero fat) without any adverse effects. They try to give you that false sense of safety so you'll buy more. Diet soda is one of the industry's great successes. It was originally billed as the solution to diabetes and overweight, but anyone can look back over the last fifty years and see that it's had no effect at all—at least no good effect. People buy it and drink it by the case, and they're still overweight and unhealthy. Aggressive marketing convinced people that at zero calories they could drink as much as they wanted, and it turned diet soda into a societal normal.

Whether you're thinking about a meal, a snack, or a dessert, avoid falling for the low-calorie trap. You can choose a real, whole food that is low-calorie by limiting the portion size. Wouldn't you rather have a 100-calorie piece of real chocolate cake than a 100-calorie, low-fat, artificially sweetened, artificially chocolate-flavored yogurt?

The all-natural trap

Natural is one of those descriptive words that isn't regulated. There is no official definition of *natural* when it's applied to a food, and *all-natural* or *100% natural* are just variations on it. But it sounds great, doesn't it? What could be healthier than something all natural? The difficulty here is that when a product is labeled *natural*, *all-natural*, or *100% natural,* it might be natural—but more frequently, it's not. So don't assume a food with one of these labels is additive-free. The only way to distinguish real from fake is to scour the label for anything else that might give it away.

The vegetarian/vegan trap

Labeling a product *vegetarian* or *vegan* automatically carries the aura of healthy.

But beware. Read the label because vegetarian just means no meat—there's nothing in that term that guarantees a lack of additives or even that a food contains vegetables. Vegetarians and vegans need to be especially vigilant because many meat substitutes contain undesirable additives, which are often required to make the product palatable. To avoid this trap, stick to real, whole vegetables, fruits, and grains and be very selective about soy-protein derivatives.

The quantity trap

We are a quantity-based society. Bigger house, more cars, more electronic gadgets, bigger big-screen TV, larger pizza, larger beer glass, bigger steak, bigger bucket of chicken, bigger strawberries: these are all things that tempt us. So it's a struggle to get ourselves to accept smaller as better. And when it comes to food we're used to large portions, so we tend to buy more to be sure we have enough. The food industry knows this and baits us with our desire for quantity through the better deal: buy this bigger package and you'll save money! But it's not a better deal if you buy the bigger package, can't use it all, and end up throwing the rest away. Or you buy the bigger package and consume it just because it's there.

You become a victim of the quantity trap when you let it trick or force you into buying more than you need—whatever the reason.

The bargain trap

Most of us are strapped for money so it's easy to become a victim of the bargain trap. If there's a sale on some food you normally eat, it won't spoil before you can consume it or you can freeze it for later, then it's a good deal. However, if the sale is only on the larger quantity package and you don't normally eat that much of the product, it's not a good deal. And keep in mind that the majority of bargains are for processed foods.

You can avoid the bargain trap by not buying things you don't need just because they're on sale. *Especially* if they are processed foods.

The coupon trap

The coupon trap is just like the bargain trap except that sometimes you can get bargains on real, whole foods. This is almost never true with coupons. I don't know if I've ever seen a coupon for fresh broccoli. I only see coupons for highly processed foods and household products.

Don't fall for the coupon trap. If you have a coupon for toothpaste or laundry soap, by all means use it. If it's for some kind of meat helper or highly sweetened yogurt or artificially flavored and colored popsicles, try to remember that's not real food.

The convenience trap

The convenience trap is probably one of the hardest to avoid. There are never enough hours in the day to get everything done, and it's tempting to cut corners with pre-prepared meals, food bars, and anything labeled *instant*. Or to hit the closest fast-food restaurant. The food industry uses this to their advantage; they know that when push comes to shove and you're short on time, you probably won't scrutinize the label—you'll just grab something and go with it. There's no doubt that these foods are convenient when you're on the run, but an apple and a small bag of whole nuts are convenient too, and they're much better for you.

Everyone needs a shortcut now and then, and that's ok (remember the 80/20 rule). But the best way to avoid the convenience trap is to gradually develop shortcuts for having real, whole foods at the ready. When you know you have a better, healthier alternative that you can throw together quickly, you won't need to settle for the industrial shortcut. There are many natural convenient alternatives.

The healthy-food-is-unsatisfying trap

Several food manufacturers use this approach to appeal to people who have just gotten sick of the barrage of faux health messages and the trendy natural approach to living.

Hormel ran a TV commercial that made fun of the all-natural trend, showing a house in a yard overgrown with weeds, a goat munching contentedly away on the roof, and a man and his wife half hidden by the overgrowth. As a curious neighbor asks the husband about it, the commercial voice chimes in with the message that you don't have to go completely natural to have natural food if you choose Hormel's Natural Choice sandwich meat. In fact, according to the label, some varieties of this product appear to be mostly additive-free. However, the overall message the commercial conveys is that pursuing a natural life makes you look ridiculous. *(youtu.be/SeYIgD2YjlE)*

Fiber One used a similar ploy in their "Turn Around Barry" commercial for Fiber One Chewy Bars. It uses the lyrics in the song to describe a man "tired of living on the taste of air," concluding with "Finally you have a manly, chocolaty snack." *(youtu.be/D5y3vkg2Pe4)* These commercials aren't aimed entirely at men. Here's one for men or women about the same product. It ends with the message "Cardboard No. Delicious Yes." *(youtu.be/wPyIfAyUL6)*

Anyway, I think you get the point. The manufacturer is positioning itself as a healthy alternative to real food based on the *common perception* that healthy food lacks taste.

The weight-loss trap

Consider the weight-loss business. You all know the formula: My name is [insert name] and I've lost [insert number] pounds with [insert name of diet program]. This statement is accompanied by before-and-after pictures, as well as a happy description of how easy it was and how great the food was. This is a strong, persuasive strategy because everyone who has a weight problem wants to believe there's some solution that will work for them—preferably one where they won't feel deprived all the time.

I doubt that the companies running these programs care whether the first time works permanently or not; as a matter of fact, they make more money if you keep re-enrolling. To avoid falling into this weight-loss trap, you'll need develop a blind eye to these ads. Continually remind yourself of a couple of facts:

- Unless you reset normal for yourself, the weight loss is not going to stick.
- Dieting is Big Business.

There are other variations on this theme. Occasionally products are marketed with a direct weight-loss appeal. The milk industry tried that with the campaign slogan "Milk helps us lose weight." Sometimes it's a celebrity association. Taylor Swift and Diet Coke; Beyonce and Pepsi. The implication is that if the "beautiful people" can consume a product and look great, you can too.

But there is no quick fix—anything that pretends to offer one just a money trap. Know the trick associations and don't fall for them. Watch out for scare tactics that might stampede you into a diet or into buying foods that imply weight loss.

If you want to find out if you've become a victim of any of these bear traps, try the next Action.

Action #4: Practice identifying the bear traps

I've described ten different marketing bear traps. Your best method of self-defense is pretty much the same for all:

- Recognize that you're a money target.
- Check out the product and the marketing claims and/or implications.
- Identify the potential trap.
- *Read the label details*.
- Evaluate the validity of the claims.
- Decide if it's a quality product or not.
- Decide if it's an appropriate quantity for you or not.
- *Refuse to be a victim of marketing—ignore the ads and focus*

on the product itself.

The most important steps in this method are in italics: *read the label details* and *refuse to be a victim of marketing*. It all comes down to how to avoid getting trapped into purchasing (and consuming) products with additives. If the product is good on its own merits—real, whole—buy it. If it's all hype and no substance, don't.

To put this into practice, choose a few common products in your food supply and answer the following questions:
- What bear trap (if any) has the company used to trap you into buying it?
- What products could you buy instead to avoid this trap?

Here's a quote attributed to Ernest Hemingway: "Every man should have a built-in crap detector operating inside him." Nothing could be better advice for beating the Marketing Machine.

PREPARE TO MAKE SMALL CHANGES

You don't have to throw everything processed out of your pantry all at once. It's easier and much less stressful to incorporate small changes and let them become normal.

Action #5: Learn the rules

Rule #1: Keep it simple

A complicated system becomes unsustainable. So when you make a change, *keep it simple.* For instance, don't try to replace one fast-food meal with a gourmet banquet. Don't suddenly try to replace all your fast-food meals with homemade ones.

Rule #2: The One-Change principle

Make one change at a time and let it become normal—that means you keep *doing the thing you changed* until you don't have to think about it anymore.

Rule #3: The Pleasure Principle

We stick mostly with habits that give us pleasure, so it's not easy to replace a bad, pleasurable habit with a better one. The book *The Brain That Changes Itself*[17] recounts how researcher Jeffrey M. Schwarz, in developing a treatment for obsessive-compulsive disorder (OCD), found that growing a new brain circuit that gives pleasure and triggers dopamine release, rewards and reinforces that new brain activity. If the new brain circuit produces more pleasure than the bad one, eventually it will replace the bad one. We adapt to change much easier when it's associated with something pleasant or enjoyable. Therefore, it's important when you substitute one food for another that you *find something that you like*. Truly healthy food is high in quality and isn't dry and tasteless, leaving you hungry an hour later.

It's possible that 80 percent of what you eat is already real, whole foods. In that case, congratulations! You can skip the rest of this how-to section and move directly into The Battle of Quantity. But to find out if you're ready, memorize the rules and take the next three Actions.

Action #6: Evaluate your food preferences

Fill out the Food Preferences chart, Evaluate Your Food Preferences in *Appendix B*. It's not a scientific assessment, but looking at your general food preferences will give you some idea of how much change lies ahead of you. It's not a gauge of what you actually eat; you might like some of the foods on the list but rarely eat them for one reason or another. What it does is suggest your *potential* for making these foods part of your personal normal.

There are four lists: Vegetables, Fruits, Grains, and Fats and you record points for each food based on the following scoring:

Description	Points
Love it!	5
Like it	4
It's ok—wouldn't refuse it but not wild about it	3
Don't know—willing to try it	2
Have never liked it, but willing to try a different preparation	1
Hate it—you couldn't pay me to eat it	0

High scores mean you have a wide variety of quality foods you already like, and that will make it easier to create whole-food meals you like. If your scores are quite low, that means you might not be very open to trying new things and changing will be more of a challenge for you. Scores above 100 for Vegetables and Fruits, 30 for Grains, and 20 for Fats put you in the easy range.

Action #7: See what you actually eat

Evaluate your *actual* eating habits by recording them on a chart. If last week was typical of the meals you usually eat, write down approximately what you ate. If it wasn't (maybe you were on vacation or there was something special going on) then choose the last week that was typical. You don't have to be too specific. Look in *Appendix B* for *See What You Actually Eat* or the online workbook, Battle of Quality, Action #7, for a sample chart. This exercise will give you a good idea of how much processed food vs. real food you already eat.

Action #8: Evaluate your current food supply

Check your pantry, fridge, and freezer and pick out twelve of your most commonly used foods. Then make a list with four columns, labeled "Whole," "In-between,", "Highly processed", and "Sugar". Based on the number of additives and/or preservatives (excluding vitamins), list each food under:

- "Whole" if it has two or fewer
- "In-between" if it has three to five
- "Highly processed" if it has more than five
- "Sugar" - number of grams

A sample chart is included in *Appendix B* and in the online workbook, Battle of Quality, Action #8. If you're unsure what ingredients are considered additives and preservatives, see *Appendix C: Additives and Preservatives*.

This Action should give you a good idea of how much processed food you commonly use and where you should start making changes.

LEARN THE RESET PROCESS

Here's a how-to for making your changes. I've used the acronym RESET because it just happens to fit and is easy to remember. It stands for **R**esearch; **E**xperiment; **S**ubstitute; **E**valuate; **T**est.

Don't let my detailed description of the RESET process make you think it's complicated. It's actually simple and intuitive; it's just difficult to quantify in words (much like trying to explain, using only words, how to tie your shoe). And after you've been through it once or twice, you won't even have to think about it.

The basic RESET process

1) **Research:** decide which food you think you should replace and find potential whole-food substitutes.
2) **Experiment:** Test your research and decide which food options you like best.
3) **Substitute:** Make your substitution in one meal or snack once a week and give yourself two to four weeks to get used to it.
4) **Evaluate:** Decide if you liked it and if it was easy enough to make that you didn't find it burdensome.
5) **Test:** If your evaluation is positive make the same substitution in other meals/snacks. If not, go back to Research and choose a different substitute.

When you have completed one substitution and it feels *normal* for you, choose another food to replace and start with the Research again.

Don't plan too far ahead; decide on one change at a time. Remember, your body will respond to your changes over time. A couple of months down the road your decision about what you think you need to change could be very different from what you think today.

In case you're thinking this will take too long, look at it this way: there are only twenty-one different meals in a week and probably fewer snacks than that, so really, there aren't that many substitutions you'll need to make to get to the 80 percent mark.

Example: Replace sweet desserts with fruit

Replacing desserts with fruit is one of the easiest examples, and you can take your time with it. The first month, choose one day of the week (Monday, for example), and replace a sweet dessert with fruit. The second month, have fruit for dessert both on Monday and on a second day (like Wednesday). The third month, add a third day of the week. There are only seven days in a week, so you can convert six of them in six

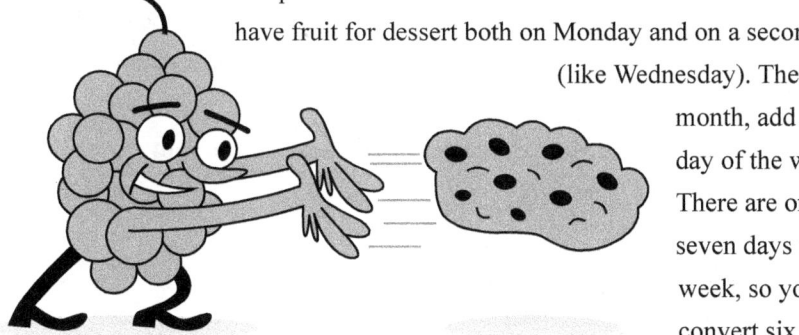

months. That seventh dinner? Nothing wrong with having a sweet dessert once a week.

Research:
- Make a list of fresh fruits that are in season and that you and your family like: grapes, apples, pears, tangerines, pineapple, berries, etc. Any fruit will do but they're always better and fresher in season, not to mention less expensive.
- Consider the potential preparation involved. For instance, grapes can just be washed and served. Same with berries. With fresh pineapple, however, you have to clean it and cut it up. You might want to slice apples and pears, and tangerines are easier to peel than oranges.
- Decide which fruit you want to start with.

Experiment:
- In this case, the switch is so simple you don't need to experiment.

Substitute:
- Choose one day of the week.
- On that day, have the fruit after dinner in place of a sweet dessert.
- Give yourself at one month to adjust to the change, but each week on the same day serve fruit. (It doesn't have to be the same fruit.)

Evaluate:
- Did you and your family like it?
- How easy was it?

Test:

If the answers to the evaluation questions was "yes":
- Keep fruit for dessert on that day of the week.
- Choose another day of the week and serve fruit instead of a sweet dessert.
- Give yourself one month to get used to the change, but if you start liking the fruit better, feel free to speed up the process by adding more fruit nights.
- You're done when you've replaced sweet desserts with fruit five or six times a week.

If the answers to the evaluation questions was "no":
- Go back to *Research* and pick a different fruit.
- Try the process again.

How to measure success—You succeed when every two months you can look back and see that you've replaced one more sweet dessert with fruit.

Example: Replace sodas with more natural beverages

I've known many people who consume eight or more cans of soda or diet soda every day. An occasional soda is not likely to harm you, but flooding your system with a product that is almost entirely artificial is not a good health decision. If you are one of those people, replacing some of those sodas should be at the top of your list. Using the RESET formula, here's an abbreviated approach.

Research: Check your local supermarket for possible alternatives, such as lightly and naturally flavored sparkling water.

Experiment: Purchase a few of these alternatives and see which ones you like best.

Substitute: Replace one standard soda with your alternative, once a day. Or if that feels too hard, even just a couple of times a week will help. The idea is that if you sneak a new one in here and there you won't feel deprived and tempted to revert.

Evaluate: Ask yourself if you liked it.

Test: If you're ok with the change, live with it for a month and then increase your replacements. If not, choose another product from your Research and try again.

Repeat this process until you've replaced most of the soda. If you can get down to two or three per week, that would be ideal. But depending on how much soda you currently consume, any reduction will give you a health benefit.

Now that you know how the process works, look over your what-you-actually-eat chart and pick something else—preferably something you think will be easy to change. With each success under your belt, the next change will be easier.

You'll find more examples in the section Help!, including:
- Replacing fast-food meals
- Replacing highly processed breads
- Replacing boxed mixes

START MAKING YOUR CHANGES

Action #9: Research

Look over your record of what you actually eat to see which processed foods you depend on most. Pushing those foods out of your diet by replacing them with real, whole foods is the key. Depending on how adventurous you feel, you can either start with the easiest item or tackle the worst offender. Keep in mind that you aren't going to make major, sudden changes in your diet, so even if you choose the worst offender, you'll phase it out a little at a time.

From my observations of what most people eat, here are some suggestions:
- Reduce your consumption of sodas.
- Replace refined white bread with whole-grain bread.
- Reduce the number of sweetened coffee drinks.
- Replace some French fries servings.
- Replace sweet desserts with fruit.
- Reduce dependence on pre-prepared frozen lunches.
- Replace sweetened yogurt.
- Reduce fast-food meals.
- Reduce your consumption of sugared cereals.

1) Choose the item you want to modify.
2) Make a short list of possible whole-food alternatives. Consider choosing

seasonally available foods, as they will taste the best. For suggestions on individual ingredients, see the *Evaluate Your Food Preferences* chart in *Appendix B*. For some full recipes, see *Whole-Food Alternatives* in *Appendix A*.

3) If you want, write your choices in the online workbook, Battle of Quality, Action #9.

Action #10: Experiment

One at a time, test out the items you found in your research and decide which you like best.

Action #11: Substitute

Choose one meal or snack on one day of the week. In that time slot every week, make your substitution. Give yourself two to four weeks to get used to the change.

Action #12: Evaluate

Ask yourself if you (and/or your family, if applicable) liked the new food and if it was easy to fix.

Action #13: Test

If you answered "yes" to both Evaluation questions:
1) Keep your current substitution.
2) Choose another meal or snack time and try your substitution there.

If you answered "no" to the Evaluation questions:
1) Go back to Action #9: Research.
2) Choosing a different substitute, follow the RESET process again.

Action #14: Repeat

Go back to Action #9: Research, choose another replacement, and follow the RESET process.

DEEPEN YOUR MIND-BODY PARTNERSHIP

Action #15: Ask your body

Begin to focus on what it is you really want to eat at each meal or snack. In the *Resetting Normal* context, you aren't locked into a particular formula. You don't have to have low-fat yogurt, dry toast, and tea for breakfast. Or a salad with chicken and low-fat dressing for lunch. When you're ready to eat breakfast in the morning, ask yourself what you really feel like eating.

At first, we are creatures of habit, but as you internalize the idea that your selection is wide open, you'll begin to listen to your body's needs. It took some time, but when I'm ready for breakfast I now know whether I feel like having cold cereal, hot cereal, an egg and toast, bacon, whole yogurt with fruit and nuts, a peanut butter sandwich, a cheese sandwich, or something else. Some days I feel like I need protein; other days I feel a need for carbs. When I listen to my body and supply what it needs, I'm satisfied for hours and I don't obsess about food.

I realize this is a vague assignment, but in *resetting normal* you should always be thinking about what your body is asking for. Until you get to at least the 60 percent whole foods level, what you think you want may have more to do with artificial cravings brought on by a processed-foods diet than with what you really need, but that will get better with time and experience.

So for how, when you get ready to eat a meal or snack, ask yourself:
- If I could have any *whole* food I wanted right now, what would it be?
- If I'm not sure what that is, can I at least choose a category: protein, carb, fat, combination?

If you've identified exactly what you want and it's available, you're in luck. If you can only identify the category, pick something in that category that's available. Either way, eat and enjoy it. Then ask yourself an hour later if you chose wisely.

AIM FOR 60 PERCENT WHOLE AND THEN MORE GRADUALLY TO 80 PERCENT

Action #16: Repeat

One change at a time, continue to replace processed foods with quality, whole foods until you've reached a point where about 80 percent of your diet consists of whole foods. Move from one RESET to the next.

Don't worry about the time this takes—you'll eventually get to that 80 percent and when you do, it will be self-sustaining.

✎ NOTES

Help!

If you've made a few replacements but aren't sure what to do to keep going or how to go about it, here are some ideas that may be helpful.

THE PATH OF LEAST RESISTANCE: CONVENIENCE FOODS

I'm not against convenience. As I've said before, the food industry responds to consumer demands and produces new products all the time. When I started writing this book, the selection of quality pre-prepared foods was abysmal. Since then the product landscape has changed, and I've seen many new products on the market that have few or no additives or preservatives.

I've seen a huge growth in the quality options now offered in the following categories:

- Frozen-food meals
- Frozen vegetable combinations
- Frozen fish
- Canned (or boxed) soups
- Canned (or boxed) broths—chicken/beef/vegetable
- Yogurts
- Cold and hot cereals
- Breads
- Refrigerated salad dressings
- Snack foods like popcorn, pretzels, crackers, and chips
- Real ice creams
- Soft drinks
- Take-out from restaurants that are more whole-food conscious
- Cookies/cakes/pies (hard to find these with real ingredients and less sugar)

If you're out to make a whole-food substitution for one of your processed standards and you can find something you like that's already prepared, use it. Just be sure to double-check the label and watch out for those marketing tricks. And prepare yourself—quality pre-packaged foods always cost more. It's one of those cases where less really is more: the less junk in the food, the more the food industry will charge for it.

SUPERMARKET SHORTCUTS

Another improvement I've noticed is that supermarkets are carrying more ready-to-make whole foods. These make meal preparation a lot easier and less time-consuming because all the ingredients are ready and all you have to do is cook them.

Some items in this category include:

- Pre-cut vegetable packs
- Pre-washed salads
- Pre-cut meats (not including lunchmeats such as salami, bologna, etc.)
- Pre-marinated, ready-to-cook meats from the butcher section
- Pre-cut fruit
- Salad bar take-home items (which are usually expensive—but a selection of specialty items you can add to your own lettuce might make your home-made salad more interesting).
- Chopped onions in the freezer section
- Chopped ginger in the freezer section or in a jar
- Pre-cleaned and cut garlic (usually in a jar of oil)

If you want to make a stir-fry you don't have to spend a half hour cutting up the vegetables. You can buy a bag of stir-fry vegetables (already cut to the right size); add some thinly sliced chicken breast, beef, or tofu; and with a wok, a little peanut oil, and soy sauce you're good to go. You can even find pre-cooked brown rice in the freezer section too.

You don't have to cut and wash salad greens anymore either; the bagged varieties are ready to eat. Avoid the ones with dressings because they have the usual processed dressing additives.

Want to make a slow cooker stew? You can combine a pack of stew-type vegetables, stewing beef cubes and one of the boxed, additive-free soups.

While you'll find that pre-cut ingredients are a little more expensive, if you're short on time and you still want to eat well, it's worth it.

WAYS TO REPLACE REFINED GRAINS

To phase out refined grains like white bread, processed sugared cereals, instant oatmeal, crackers, pasta, and so on, you have to get familiar with whole grains—what they are, how to prepare them, and how they taste. The only way to do that is to do a little research then experiment. Some you may like right away, some you might come to like over time, and of course, some you might not like at all. Whole-grain pastas have come a long way from original attempts and most supermarkets carry some varieties now.

Whole grains are wonderful for breads and side dishes, but what about using wholewheat flour for cookies and pastries? Actually, I don't. Surprised? I went down this path years ago and tried making cookies and pastries with whole-wheat flour, finally concluding that I would rather have one (butter, unbleached white flour, eggs, sugar, etc.) cookie/cake/pastry once in a while and enjoy it than have many of the whole-wheat variety. Whole wheat lends a denser texture and a taste that may override the subtle flavors in pastries.

Remember the 80/20 rule? For me this falls under the 20 percent. I don't eat these kinds of foods often, but when I do I want to enjoy one for what it is. I have a fantastic recipe for a fresh raspberry chiffon cake with a vanilla-cream filling that requires using cake flour, which is even more refined than usual all-purpose flour. It's complicated and time-consuming, so I only make it a couple times a year. So do I worry about eating it? Not a bit.

WAYS TO ADD WHOLE VEGETABLES

The brain-dead simple way to add more vegetables to your diet is just to eat a larger portion. A little less pasta or bread and a little more salad, string beans, or broccoli. Don't start out by doubling it; just serve yourself a little bit more. You can also serve two kinds of vegetables instead of one and take a little of each. But for some other ideas, see *Appendix A: Whole-Food Alternatives*.

WAYS TO REPLACE SUGAR

One of the primary ways to replace sugar is to *Fight Sugar with Fat*!
What?

Most experts will just warn you not to eat the sugar in the first place, or to choose something supposedly healthier like fat-free yogurt or veggies or maybe a protein bar. But that doesn't always work. Usually what happens is that you eat the healthier alternative, are still not satisfied, and end up eating something much worse anyway. At least that's always what happened to me.

I distinctly remember having the sugar problem. My most vivid memory is that when someone would bring donuts to work, I'd try to be good and eat only a small piece (one-quarter of the donut). I'd go back to my desk, and within ten minutes I'd become ravenously hungry. I always went back for the rest of the donut, and I admit, if it weren't that I would've been totally embarrassed, I would've eaten two or three more.

Now I have a different solution, based on my *Resetting Normal* experiences. I came to realize that many times, when I craved something sweet, either I was sleep-deprived or what I really needed was something with fat. But because fat was officially forbidden, I'd try to substitute something low-fat. This led me to eat veggies or fruit, then when I was still hungry, to eat some kind of reduced-fat muffin. The problem with this approach is that it takes less (calorically) of something high in fat to fill you up than of something low in fat. *The closer a food is to 100 percent fat, the less of it you can eat.* Once you throw refined carbs into the mix, it changes everything—thus the problem of overeating with foods like mac and cheese, donuts, pizza, and so on.

Here's what I mean.

Calorie comparison #1:
- Calories in a quarter cup of butter or vegetable oil: approximately 600
- Calories in eight ounces of cheddar cheese (a half pound): approximately 800
- Calories in a medium-size Dairy Queen Blizzard: approximately 800

I don't know about you, but I don't know anyone who could eat an entire quarter cup of butter or oil by itself in one sitting (without getting sick). I also don't know of many people who could comfortably down a half pound of cheese. But I do know people who can eat a medium-size Dairy Queen Blizzard in one sitting—even after a hamburger lunch. There's no sugar in the butter, vegetable oil or cheese, but the Blizzard has a whopping eighty-four grams, which equates to seven tablespoons or almost a half cup. That's a lot of sugar to load into your system at one time.

Calorie comparison #2:
- Calories in two fried eggs: approximately 200
- Calories in one of those giant, low-fat muffins that have become standard: approximately 450

These are ordinary breakfast items, but the two eggs have no sugar and they'll satisfy hunger for hours. The muffin is loaded with refined flour, sugar and flavorings, will not last you as long and it has more than twice the calories.

Calorie comparison #3:

I finally learned from experience that a small, high-fat snack would quiet my appetite for several hours at least, and I'd consume fewer calories that way than if I tried to fill up on low-fat food and failed. Consider, instead of that low-fat 450 calorie muffin:

- Two ounces of cheese and two crackers (about 250 calories)
- Two ounces of cheese and a small apple (about 250 calories)
- Half a peanut butter sandwich (with two tablespoons of peanut butter, about 300 calories)

I'm not suggesting you eat a high-fat diet overall, but when you're faced with a choice between some refined sweet thing and something with fat or oil, choose the fat because it will kill your appetite quicker than anything else. I once had an eggplant lunch in an Asian restaurant and it had so much oil in it that I wasn't hungry until seven hours later. As a matter of fact, I didn't even want to *think* about eating before then.

Other ways to replace sugar are:
- Eat fruit for dessert and snacks.
- Add whole milk or half and half to coffee and gradually reduce the sweetener.
- Drink less fruit juice—eat the whole fruit and drink water.
- Counter sweet office snacks by occasionally bringing in artisan bread and cheese.

Just remember: try these replacements gradually, not all at once.

WAYS TO USE FATS AND OILS RESPONSIBLY

There's a huge war being raged against fat, but believe it or not, there are options besides supposedly trans-fat-free margarine and canola oil. The oils I use most often are extra virgin olive oil, butter and mayonnaise, flax oil, peanut oil, corn oil, and coconut oil. For those of you who are deathly afraid of butter, mayonnaise, and sour cream, you can use less by mixing them with vegetable oils. I still believe real fat is better than reduced-fat varieties because those have undesirable fillers and additives.

It's quite possible to use fats and oils responsibly. I don't worry about how much fat or oil I use anymore. But that's because I've learned that a little goes a long way, and I don't eat fried foods very often. I also use grass-fed meats whenever I can afford them. Because of that my overall consumption of fat is pretty low. Fat is self-limiting if you aren't combining it with sugar or refined carbohydrates. If I happen to use more oil, it just keeps me full for a longer time so I'm not constantly snacking.

For those of you worried about saturated fat, you can still use butter and real mayonnaise—just use less of it. And you can add flavor to extra-lean meats by adding olive oil. If your ground beef is so lean it makes a dry burger, try mixing in some olive oil when making the patties; it will enhance the flavor and the texture.

Solve the salad dressing problem. What is the salad dressing problem? It doesn't take much dressing to make a salad taste good—basically, it should be just enough to lightly coat the ingredients. Getting this right is easy. All it requires is a large bowl and a couple of spoons or forks.

At home, it's just a matter of experimenting to find out how much dressing works. When you make a salad, choose a bowl much bigger than the amount of salad, add a little dressing, and toss lightly until it's evenly distributed. When you first start tossing, it may not seem like enough dressing, but keep going—it takes at least fifteen or twenty tosses to get the job done. And you may be surprised at how little dressing it takes. You shouldn't end up with pools of dressing in the bottom of the bowl. I find that for about three cups of salad, a dressing that uses only one tablespoon of olive oil, some vinegar, mustard and spices is sufficient. If you have a family where everyone likes a different kind of dressing, give each person a bowl big enough for tossing and let them have fun.

At a restaurant, it's almost impossible. A higher-end restaurant will have your salad already dressed with the chef's idea of how much is appropriate. In my experience, mid-level restaurants tend to use too much dressing (with questionable ingredients). There, your best option is to ask for it on the side and drizzle as best as you can. Worse yet are the salad bars. There you get a small plate (to discourage you from taking very much, no doubt) and no chance of any way to toss it.

All in all, it isn't hard to get used to a salad with just enough dressing to make it taste perfect; it's a matter of adjusting your expectations. I suggest starting with a small amount, toss and test, and add a little more if you need to. Try to find the least amount you need to enhance your salad.

USING REAL CHEESE

If you're eating foods that are made with processed cheese or reduced-fat cheese (like boxed mac and cheese or a creamy pasta dish) you're probably used to the creamy texture from the additives. To make an equivalent creamy dish from real cheese, simply combine real cheddar cheese and real Monterey Jack in your recipe. The jack cheese will give it the creamy texture you're used to.

To reiterate, if you're worried about saturated fat, you can still use real cheese—just use less of it.

WAYS TO REPLACE BOXED MIXES

There's no doubt that boxed mixes are convenient. But the health consequences aren't. Anything you can do to reduce your consumption of them is to your benefit.

Sweet stuff. One of the reasons we eat too many cookies, cakes, pies, and pastries is that it's convenient to buy them or make them from a boxed mix. Yes, it takes more time and effort to make them from scratch, but that's a good thing because it means you'll think twice before doing it, and the end result is that you'll eat fewer of them. Our metabolism is not designed to handle those highly processed foods on a daily basis.

That doesn't mean you have to go cold turkey and quit them all at once. But there are some super-simple from-scratch recipes available. I have a couple of standbys where I just throw all the ingredients in a bowl, beat the heck out of them, pour the batter into a pan, and bake—a wonderful solution to the problem where your kid tells you at 8:00 p.m. that he or she needs something to take to school the next day. See *Appendix A: Whole-Food Alternatives* for some easy ideas.

Dinner helpers. Boxed dinner helpers may save some time, but not that much when you have the right ingredients on hand. The only convenience the box offers is the seasoning and pre-cooked carb filler (pasta, rice, etc.); you still have to cook the meat. To make the equivalent without the box, start with the carb. If you cook the dry form, pasta takes only about fifteen minutes so if you do that first thing, it will be ready when the meat is. If you keep some brown rice handy in the freezer, just defrost it and throw it in. And with a few basic seasonings you can create a great-tasting dish without all the additives and preservatives.

For basic lists of ingredients to keep on hand for making your own sweets and dinners, see *Appendix A: Whole-Food Alternatives.*

WAYS TO MAKE PREPARATION EASIER AND SHORTER

I save myself a lot of time by making more than I need and freezing the extra for future use. However, that does require freezer space. If you have a separate freezer or a refrigerator with a large freezer, that can work for you. The one thing you need to make this successful is a good freezer label.

Another way is to use a slow cooker See *Appendix A: Whole-Food Alternatives* for recommendations on choosing cookbooks and recipes.

HOW TO REBALANCE YOUR MEALS

Growing up in the 1950s, we were taught to create balanced lunches or dinners by combining a protein, a vegetable, a starch, and something sweet. I still use this plan today because it provides interesting, varied meals and covers all the nutritional bases. One exception: back then, "something sweet" usually meant cookies, cake, or pie, and I serve fruit instead. Proteins include meat, eggs, poultry, soy, or something similar. A qualifying vegetable is usually green or yellow (salad, broccoli, summer squash, etc.), and a starch includes anything made from grains or vegetables (potatoes, carrots, peas, winter squash, etc).

It isn't hard to do this. In a way, it makes everything easier because you don't have to sort through all possibilities, you just pick one from each of those categories. It helps you stay away from monotonous, dense meals. If you're going to have pasta for dinner, you don't need bread—complement it with a salad instead. If you serve potatoes, don't serve corn. And don't serve just a protein with a green vegetable because grain-based foods help fill you up. This a problem with many restaurant lunches—you can order the salad with grilled chicken, but (for me, at least) this isn't satisfying without a bit of bread to go with it. This balance technique even works with convenience meals. Add a salad to a pizza dinner and you're good to go.

Why this replacement process works

HOW I CHANGED WHEN I RESET NORMAL

Except for a few specific examples, you may have noticed that I haven't told you what I eat now that I've reset my normal. That's intentional because I don't want you to start projecting my changes into your potential future. Your eating patterns may end up being very different from mine. It's a personal journey.

When I started my journey, I didn't have a specific goal other than to stop my crazy dieting. I didn't say things like, "I'm going to give up donuts forever," "I will only eat fruit for dessert," "I will only let myself eat pizza once every couple of months," "I will give up eating anything with sugar in it," "I will only eat whole-wheat pasta," or "I will eat vegetables for lunch every day."

What happened to me evolved over time (several years, and it's still changing even now). I will occasionally eat a donut, but they're not a temptation anymore, especially the ones drowned in sugar icing. I do prefer fruit for dessert. I don't crave pizza and we probably have it only once every couple of months. I'm ok with a little sugar, but I don't like anything overly sweet; I'm not a fan of chocolate-chip cookies anymore (I used to easily scarf down a dozen) or the super-sweet bakery cakes and pies. I will eat any kind of pasta, but prefer the whole-wheat varieties. And I do like to have a vegetable soup or stew or salad for lunch (sometimes with some protein, sometimes without). One of the best side effects of all the changes is that when I eat what I want (selecting from real, whole foods), I'm satisfied and I can go about my business without obsessing over the next snack or meal.

That just skims the surface of my changes—there have been many, many more. But the important point is that *I did not set out to make any of them specifically*. I did not start out to get to a specific dietary place; I just ended up where I am because my journey took me there. I'd get to one place by making gradual changes and as that place became comfortable (normal), I stayed there. I would never, ever in a million years have predicted that I'd be where I am now and feel comfortable and natural with it. This should be reassuring for you, as it demonstrates that *Resetting Normal* does not require you to force yourself to eat, avoid, or do anything that's so far out of your normal you can't handle it easily.

DON'T FALL FOR THE FALLACY OF EXTRAPOLATION

My experience also demonstrates that you shouldn't fall for what I call the Fallacy of Extrapolation. We all try to predict what the future will be based on our current and past experiences. That may seem logical but it does not account for random changes that happen along the way. Nothing about life is linear; it never marches on in a straight line.

So you may be sitting on your sofa reading this book and thinking that you love chocolate so much, if there's ever a tray of brownies on the counter, you will *always* be tempted to eat them all. You cannot imagine *not* wanting those brownies or eating just one and being satisfied. You might believe that no matter what, if you open a bag of potato chips, you'll eat your way through the whole thing. You might be convinced that if you had a choice between grapes and cheesecake for dessert, you would *always* take the cheesecake. Maybe you can't imagine turning down a second helping of mashed potatoes and gravy, or choosing roast chicken over fried. And surely, you can't imagine looking at a donut and saying, "Meh … no thanks."

But that's because it's the way you are *now*—what your normal is now. What you have to realize is that when you change what you eat, you also change your response to food—your body undergoes *physical changes* in response to the food you give it. And *from where you are now, you have no way of knowing how those changes will affect you.*

What I claim is not without precedent. Millions of people can and do change their food preferences all the time.

How do you make that happen?
- Sometimes you might just try something different, maybe in a different environment or situation and suddenly it's a totally different experience.
- Sometimes, it's a matter of trying a food prepared differently.
- Sometimes it's a matter of getting accustomed (normalized) to something different over time.
- Sometimes a medical condition will compel you to change—fear is a powerful motivator.

Now, some of your preferences may never change. If you have strong aversions to certain types of foods, it's unlikely you'll start to love them. If you really, really hate the taste and/or texture of fish (or some other food), you probably aren't going to become a convert, either overnight or over time. But the good news is that's ok because there's such a wide variety of real, whole foods, you can avoid some without handicapping your health. I know someone who doesn't like cauliflower at all, but he's fine with broccoli, so who cares? Lots of people hate Brussels sprouts—if that's you, don't eat them. There are plenty of alternatives.

MY THEORIES

There are lots of theories circulating today about why we can't lose weight, and why we are attracted to foods high in sugar and fat. There's also much scientific study devoted to the topic. This research is important, but it focuses on the micro level: the molecular components and how they work in the metabolism and brain. It's slow, tedious work and it's likely to go on for a long time before anything definitive comes from it.

In the meantime, I take a macro view, which is much simpler. *We are what we eat*: everything we eat is broken down into molecules and mysteriously processed by our metabolism for energy, thought processes and cell building and repair. This process has worked for the most part since the dawn of mankind, so even if some things do occasionally go wrong, if we eat what we've been evolved (or designed) to, *most everything* should work correctly. If something isn't working correctly, we shouldn't immediately jump to the conclusion that we're broken and we need drugs to fix it. In the last couple of centuries we've been eating in ways that are entirely new to our metabolic system, so it's no wonder things have gone haywire. Our first line of rescue should be to correct what we're eating. If that fixes the problem, we're done. If not, *then* it's time to look at something more drastic.

Based on that assumption, I have two theories about why and how changing what we eat to real, whole foods becomes easier over time and allows us to reset normal.

Theory #1

The current Western style of eating does not provide your metabolism with all the elements it needs—thus spawning wild cravings, hunger, inability to control quantity, lack of energy, mood swings, depression, and a host of other problems. When you switch to real, whole foods your body gradually goes through a healing process. It might take a year or two; cellular repair takes time. As your body becomes able to function and repair itself more effectively and efficiently, those undesirable symptoms disappear and you can go without food for longer periods of time. When your body has what it needs to operate at a cellular level, it stops bugging you.

Theory #2

There's been a lot of research lately on the effect of gut bacteria that inhabit our intestinal tract and help us digest food. One line of thought in this arena is that transplanting some of the gut bacteria from a thin person's colony into a fat person's colony will help the fat person lose weight. But this assumes that overweight people can't cultivate their own anti-fat bacteria.

I believe the type of bacteria inhabiting someone's gut is directly related to *what they eat*, and the type of bacteria inhabiting someone's gut influences what that person *wants to eat*. In other words, the colony of gut bacteria has evolved to live on whatever the person feeds it. It naturally wants to continue to survive, so it affects metabolic processes that drive the person to feed it more of the same.

What kind of gut bacteria do you cultivate when you drink soda (regular or diet), consume a lot of sugar and refined carbohydrates, and continually bombard it with chemically processed additives like artificial flavors and colors, modified food starch, and preservatives? You get the kind that thrives on junk and wants more. The kind that makes you unable to control your appetite, and consequently makes you gain weight.

Now suppose you gradually start changing what you eat to real, whole foods. At first, nothing noticeable happens. But then, over time, a colony of gut bacteria that thrives on those foods begins to grow, and it wants to survive. So it manipulates your metabolism in such a way that you begin to want more and more of those healthy foods. As you phase out the junk foods, the old, bad colony of gut bacteria shrinks, and with it, your cravings for that kind of food.

How these theories can help you

Regardless of whether you give credence to any of my theories, it's an observable phenomenon that people can and do change their food preferences over time. It also gets easier over time, which means there must be some internal changes going on there. Just because you like or don't like certain foods this very moment doesn't mean it will always remain that way. Don't get it into your head that at the end of the *Resetting Normal* road you can never have brownies or chocolate-chip cookies. That's not how this works.

This is how it *does* work. You make a small change. Your body responds to that change. You make another change. Your body responds to that change. You make still another change and your body responds to that one, and so on. With each iteration of change and response, the base set of conditions in your body evolves—which in turn makes the next change easier.

The power of this solution is in *changing your preferences*. By the time you get to the fifth or tenth or hundredth change in this process, your body's metabolism is working differently. And guess what? That's when your *preferences* change. If you *prefer* a lighter dish over a heavy one; if you *prefer* whole-wheat bread to white; if you *prefer* fresh fruit to cookies for dessert; if you *prefer* water to soda—then there is no choice conflict, no fight over whether to eat the bad one or not. You get to eat what you want because *what you want now is good for you.*

Don't try to imagine what your food banquet will be like in the future based on what it is today. Heraclitus was a Greek philosopher and probably the first to verbalize the concept that the only constant in life is change. Embrace the change and the potential it offers.

Measuring Success

As you progress, measure your success by looking back two months. If you've replaced two or three processed foods regularly with an equivalent whole food that you like, and you've kept that substitution, you're succeeding.

As these substitutions accumulate, try to estimate whether you've reached the point where about 50-60 percent of your weekly food consumption is whole. At that point, cravings triggered by processed, refined foods should be diminished enough that you can start to think about *how much* you eat. Feel free to take the next step: you don't have to get all the way to 80 percent before starting The Battle of Quantity.

NOTES

CHAPTER 10
THE BATTLE OF QUANTITY
The Context

WHAT IS THE BATTLE OF QUANTITY?

We live in a society that thinks more is better. More clothes, more jewelry, more cars, more travel, more food, more whatever. We face pressure from within ourselves, our social circles, and our capitalist economy to consume more of everything. As long as you have the money to pay for them, buying more products is not necessarily a bad thing; I can't think of any downsides to having more jewelry. But food is different—because an excess of it is a driver of yo-yobesity and can harm or even kill you. The Battle of Quantity is a fight against this excess.

WHY IS IT SO IMPORTANT?

There's a lot to be said for everything in moderation when it comes to your body. Too much of anything is not healthy. Too much exercise can damage muscles and bones. Too much alcohol will damage your liver. Too much sugar will overload your pancreas. Too many Brazil nuts will deliver a toxic dose of the mineral selenium. Even too much of a vegetable such as bok choy can kill you (if you eat it raw). And at the other end of the spectrum, too little of some things is not healthy. Too little vitamin C, and you get scurvy. Too little vitamin

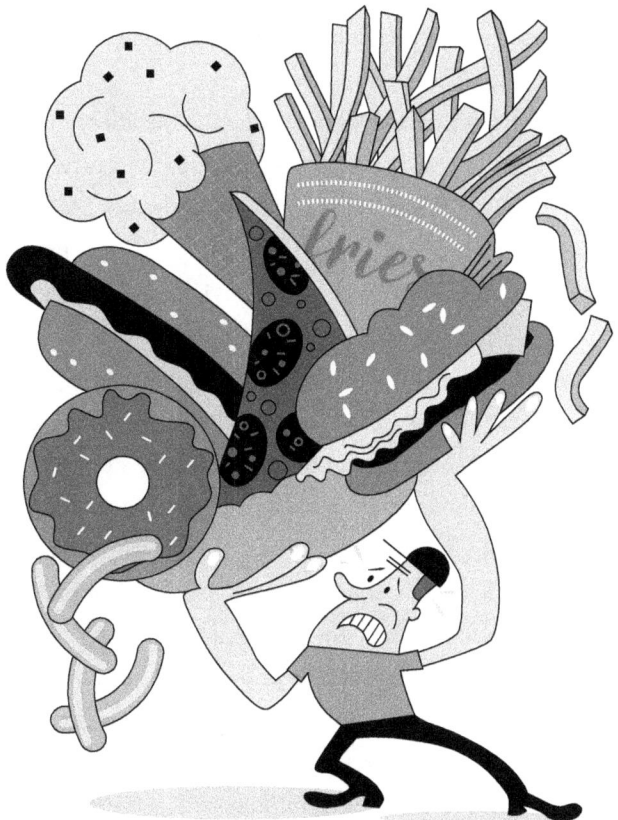

D and calcium, and children get rickets. Too little fiber results in constipation. Too little water will impact all bodily functions.

When your health is at stake it's important to pay attention to this quantity thing and get a handle on it.

WHAT MAKES IT SO DIFFICULT TO CONTROL OVEREATING?

I've already talked about the external forces: experts telling us what, when, and how much to eat; the power of marketing; the power of the social normal; and other factors. But there are internal forces at work as well.

Theories about our biology

The current popular theory on why we overeat is that we evolved in an environment where the food supply wasn't steady. Consequently, we have genes that push us to gorge on food whenever we can to build up fat reserves so that we can survive famines. The claim is that while that survival strategy worked for us in early human history, it's backfiring on us today because we don't have famines anymore, at least in the industrial world. Quite the opposite: we have too much food and our genes haven't adapted to this new environmental feast. We simply can't help ourselves from eating to excess when we can.

I'm not in a position to argue whether this theory is correct or not, but not everyone exhibits this stockpiling behavior. Consequently, I propose an additional theory.

We have to eat to survive and up until the last hundred years or so, we did so by personally hunting, gathering, farming by hand, preparing, and preserving food from raw materials. This level of activity required a substantial amount of energy, which in turn required a substantial amount of food—in its whole form—and we have evolved a digestive apparatus to support those needs. If you look at a diagram of the digestive system, you can see that it takes up a significant amount of space inside the body. And part of that system—the stomach—is even expandable. This design allowed our ancestors to stuff in the food, filling up the space to feel full and satisfied, then go about their daily activities while the system did its processing.

Now, all that biological machinery worked just fine until the advent of technological automation. With automation, we no longer have to expend great amounts of energy just to survive. Compared to the calories that people once required, our requirement is abysmally small. Consequently, our true requirement for food is small.

But wait—this has created a huge disconnect. While our energy requirements for survival shrank dramatically, our digestive system did not. We may not need it, but we still have the capacity to process a large amount of food. Our stomachs demand that we fill them up, so we do. Not only that, they want something to keep them busy for a while; they used to take hours to digest their contents. But with what we feed them now (refined, processed foods), our stomachs can be done with that task in minutes. Then there's nothing left for them to do but get bored and bug us to eat more.

Thus we have the conditions for a perfect storm of conflict between demand and supply:

DEMAND	SUPPLY
Small energy requirement	Excess energy supply
Large physical capacity designed for the bulk of whole foods	Refined foods with little bulk
Digestive system designed to process food slowly, providing a steady energy supply that controls hunger	Refined food that is processed fast, providing an erratic energy supply that fuels hunger

Essentially, we're shoveling the wrong kind of fuel into the system then wondering why it isn't working properly.

It may be that a combination of these theories drives our overeating, but the genetic theory implies there's no possible solution, while my theory allows you to address the problem by simply providing your digestive system with the kind of fuel it was designed for. Switching to the right kind of fuel was what The Battle of Quality was all about. If you've mostly won that battle, you'll be prepared to tackle the other reasons we overeat. Even so, winning The Battle of Quantity is the most difficult of all.

Our broken appestat

Another reason we have trouble controlling how much we eat is that too much outside interference has left us with broken appestats. We don't start out that way; eating means survival so unless you have some genetic metabolic defect, when you're born you respond to your signals of hunger and fullness. When a baby is hungry, it cries. When it's full, it sleeps. That's its built-in appestat at work—the internal appetite-control mechanism. But as the child grows, we (parents) fix that, don't we? We have some preconceived notion about how much and when children should eat, and if they don't want to comply we apply pressure until they do.

And that's where it all starts. "Johnny, you have to sit there until you finish your dinner." "Mary, you can't have any dessert unless you eat all your peas." "Scott, you can't go out to play unless you eat lunch." Obviously, children need guidance—I had three, so I know—but in retrospect, I now see how I overplayed this aspect of parenting, and even as adults, my kids suffer the consequences. Forcing kids to eat when they're not hungry is the first blow against their built-in appestat.

Add to that: family interactions. How many of us have eaten something we didn't want or were too full to eat, just so we didn't insult the person who made it? "No seconds for you, Zack? I guess you don't like it very much." "There's just one piece of chicken left—someone please eat it so I don't have to throw it out." "You must have some—Aunt Beth made that especially for you." We learn that we have to eat to please others. Strike another blow against the built-in appestat.

Add to that: a diet of refined, processed foods. Too much sugar, not enough bulk, not enough nutrition, but lots of calories. No way for your body to tell whether it's full or not. The number of calories should make the appestat point to full, but the lack of bulk and nutritional elements makes it point to hungry. Strike another blow against the built-in appestat.

Add to that: a covey of experts telling us what, when and how much to eat. This one is pretty much the death knell. By this time, we're so disconnected from our appestat, we don't even realize we have one. We listen to the experts even when our body tries to tell us the advice is wrong. Just like our parents did to us, we try to find a way to make our body comply. Final blow to the built-in appestat.

I've been through all the above scenarios, and I seriously thought for most of my life that my appestat was defective. I assumed that since I always gained weight, my appetite must be naturally greater than my metabolism and there was nothing I could do about it. But I was wrong. *My appestat was not defective—it was simply suppressed.* Now that I've reactivated it, it's working just fine. The Battle of Quantity is all about how you can fix yours.

NOTES

The Challenges

THE GOLDILOCKS QUEST

The Context

Why Goldilocks?

Just in case you never read the childhood story of *Goldilocks and the Three Bears*, here's a brief synopsis:

> *A little girl named Goldilocks is wandering through the woods when she comes across the home of three bears: Momma Bear, Papa Bear, and Baby Bear. The three bears were out for a walk and had left their bowls of porridge on the table to cool. Goldilocks enters their home and sees the bowls of porridge. She tastes one and finds it too hot, then the next one and finds it too cold, and finally the third, which is just right so she eats it all up. Then she tries out their chairs. The first one is too big, the second is also too big, and the third one is just right—but when she sits in it, it breaks. Finally she tries out their beds. The first is too hard, the second is too soft, and the third one is just right, so she falls asleep in it. The bears, of course, return while she's sleeping. She wakes up, gets scared, and runs home.*

The Goldilocks Quest is a metaphor for the essence of The Battle of Quantity because it's the search for the quantity of food that's just right for you. Not the quantity that someone else tells you is right, but the quantity that you, yourself, *know* is right because you can feel it.

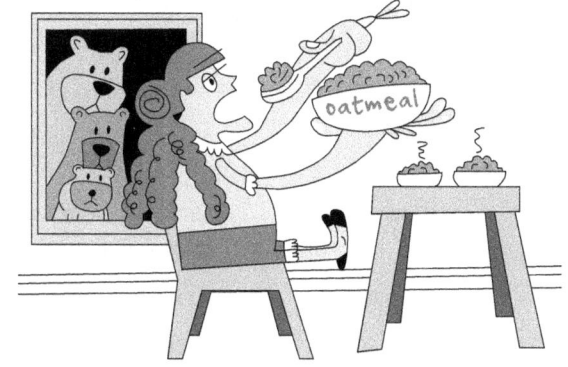

Now some people don't have a problem with how much to eat. I'm sure you've met a few. They're the ones who leave food on their plates, who might respond to an invitation to lunch with, "I'm going to go later. I'm not hungry yet." Those of us who do have a problem judging how much to eat are left wondering, "Why can't I be like that?" So, the challenge is, how can you become like that? How do you find and accept your Goldilocks feeling?

Until you experience it firsthand, the best way I can describe this Goldilocks feeling is from my own experience. Starting about an hour after I've eaten a meal and extending for two or three hours, my stomach feels perfect. Not too full, not at all hungry, just right. Completely satisfied. A warm glow permeates my torso, as if my system is producing a perfect, steady flow of energy.

The first time I experienced it was serendipitous. I had eaten a breakfast of fruit, one egg, one piece of bacon, a piece of whole-wheat toast with a little jam, and some coffee. I don't remember exactly what I was doing an hour after I ate, but I do remember that I felt so good that I noticed it. It was one of those, "Whoa—what's going on here?" moments. I thought, "That must have been a perfect breakfast. I'm not too full and I'm not hungry. I just feel absolutely great!" And that was the beginning of my Goldilocks Quest—the search for other food combinations and meals in the right quantity that would produce the same effect.

It wasn't a straightforward journey because there was a lot of interference: outside influences, entrenched perceptions, and old habits, to mention a few. But eventually I did figure out how to hit the sweet spot close enough and often enough, I no longer needed anyone else to tell me how much to eat and I'm not tempted to eat more than is comfortable for me.

And that's the point. If someone else tells you that you should eat only half a cup of mac and cheese, that has a whole different psychological effect than if you know from personal experience that half a cup of mac and cheese makes you feel just right. You'll fight the former but you'll enjoy the latter. Dieting according to someone else's specifications requires willpower. Eating what makes you feel good does not. And that empowers you.

The objective

The Goldilocks Quest will negate the need for tracking calories. Based on your body's metabolic state, you'll be able to discern what and how much to eat. Humankind's internal appestat has done this for thousands of years, and it's good at it. Overriding it by tracking calories and forcing it to submit to some random external algorithm is part of the reason we've lost control. The daily calorie limit is just a laboratory average. Your energy uses vary continuously and when you try to stick to one number, you are forcing a dynamic system into a static mode.

Consider comparing it to the speed of a car. What if someone added up all the speed limits throughout the country, calculated the average, then dictated that everyone should drive at that average speed all the time, no matter the circumstances.

Sounds insane, doesn't it? That speed would be too slow for the freeway and too fast for a school zone or busy intersection. And what about starting up or slowing down? It would be absurd. Yet, we're expected to make our bodies function under the same kind of formula.

There's no reason that, with a little practice, you can't revive your own personal appestat. Find your starting point and work through some of the assignments. These are not one-time assignments; they're tools you can use over and over in various ways to help you find your Goldilocks Quantity.

The best defense against overeating is being full *and satisfied* (you can be full and not satisfied), and the best way to learn how to get to that point is to pursue The Goldilocks Quest.

Action #1: Find a starting point

Give some thought to an everyday, *quality* (whole foods) meal you've had that you really enjoyed and that kept you satisfied for hours. If you can't think of one that completely fits that description, try to think of one that's close. Do not consider calories, fat, carbs, or any other value for your selection. It should be strictly based on something of *quality* that you *like*.

Once you have that meal in mind, you have your Goldilocks benchmark. You might want to write it down in your copy of the workbook.

Action #2: Employ a feedback loop

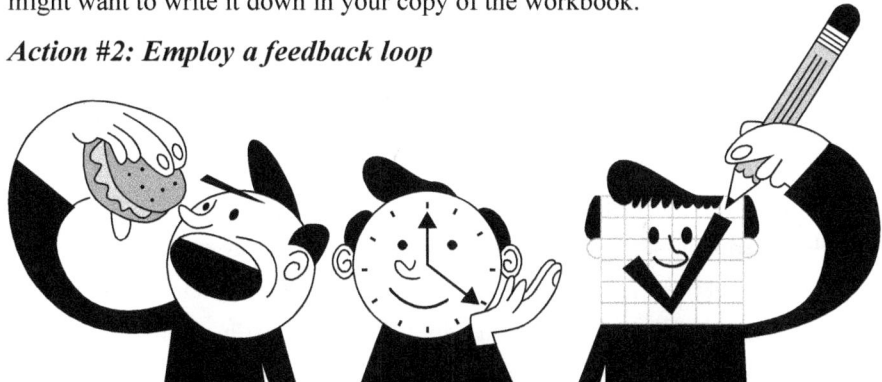

Eat a snack or meal, noting what it was and how much you ate. An hour later, using your benchmark, evaluate your appetite comfort level: hungry again, just right, or too full. If it isn't just right, the next time you eat that particular snack or meal, make adjustments by eating more or less of it.

The goal of this tool is to help you get a sense of just how much food makes you feel good and satisfied for some hours. Getting into that state frees your mind from obsession over when you can eat again and allows you to engage in something more productive. Don't expect to achieve the Goldilocks feeling with every meal you eat, but just looking for it will help you begin to reactivate your own internal appestat.

Here's an example of quantity feedback:

One day I improvised a lunch. I grabbed a half cup brown rice, one small can of tuna packed in olive oil, one small tomato, and a half teaspoon seasoning. As a last thought, I grabbed a leftover half an avocado. At work, I made a salad from those items and ate it all. But then, an hour later, I felt totally stuffed and I realized that the last-minute addition of half an avocado was overload. So the next time I considered adding avocado to a lunch I only used a small slice, or I left it out altogether. Since then I've associated small amounts of avocado on top of a meal with a feeling of being full and satisfied. But I had to experience it myself before I could make that association for the future.

You might want to make some notes about your discoveries for future reference. When you do feel "just right" after a meal, make a note that it's one of your Goldilocks meals and file it in your "proven" meal/snack repertoire in the workbook. Try out other meals, one at a time. You don't have to do this with everything you eat, but you should collect about five Goldilocks meals.

Here are a few tips:

Learn to deal with the half-a-fruit-problem. Plant breeding over the centuries has resulted in some varieties of fruit that are huge—too large for one serving. Cutting one piece in half doesn't seem right because the half that's left starts to look ugly pretty quickly. I resisted half-fruit portions for years because of that, but I've finally come to terms with it. If it's an apple that's too large for me, I will now cut it in half, wrap half in plastic and store it in the refrigerator. Yes, the sides get brown, but that's only superficial—they can be trimmed off. Bananas are even worse, but now I do that too—I cut them in half and wrap the open end. When I want the other half, I trim off the ugly part. I don't like it but I do it because sometimes a whole banana is more than I want. Don't feel compelled to eat a whole fruit if you find you're getting full.

Embrace serendipity. Sometimes you discover the right amount simply by accident. When I was working I usually had all the parts of my lunch ready to go, but one day I forgot to pack one of the items. When I ate what I did pack, though, I realized that it was enough; I didn't really need what I *thought* I was going to need.

Action #3: Try quality instead of quantity

When you're hungry, the type of food you select is sometimes more important than the quantity. It's better to choose foods that satisfy. A cup of raw veggies is fine if that's what you want and what feels good to you at the moment. It certainly has the volume to fill up your stomach. But if you eat that and you're still hungry, it wasn't volume that you needed—it was something else. That something else could be protein, fat, or maybe a different kind of carbohydrate.

Pick a meal or snack and try to figure out what you really want. Give yourself permission to experiment. Instead of choosing based on calories, fat, or carbs, focus on whole-foods quality and satisfaction. Wait an hour. If you're still hungry, it probably wasn't what you needed. Ask yourself what you might have eaten instead that would've done the trick. Get comfortable with the idea that you don't have to stuff yourself because you can eat more later.

The Goldilocks Quest is about learning to get in touch with your body so you can figure out what you really need to eat. With practice you become a better judge of what works and what doesn't. *Always ask yourself what you feel like eating, if anything.*

Action #4: Try to choose the right foods at the right time

Because we have food available to us 24/7, sometimes we eat for the wrong reasons. I found that getting rid of the psychological baggage of dieting in the Battle of the Mind cleared up my emotional eating problems. But there were still other scenarios where I felt driven to eat even though I wasn't hungry.

Don't eat something just because you think you're supposed to. I had to learn to listen to my stomach instead of outside recommendations. If you're not hungry first thing in the morning, eat later when you are. Maybe you ate too much the night before and your body is still processing it. Don't be constrained by *what* you think you're supposed to eat either. Breakfast doesn't have to be eggs, toast, cereal, or yogurt. If you want cereal, eat cereal. If you want an egg, eat an egg. But if you have a craving for a hamburger, eat that. If you want a peanut butter sandwich, eat one.

Recognize boredom. Another scenario was that sometimes I wanted to eat even though I wasn't hungry. One of the reasons was boredom. The other was a need to fill time while waiting for something. I learned to combat this problem with a simple technique. First, I asked myself if I was really hungry or if I just felt antsy—a need to be doing something.

If I was hungry, then it was time for a snack that would satisfy. That might be nuts, cheese, peanut butter and crackers, hummus, or the like. I could eat that and be done with it—hunger begone!

If it was the latter, I found the answer was eating something I could chew on that wasn't heavily filling. If you like chewing gum, this would be the time for that. It wasn't the answer for me because I don't like chewing gum. Instead I found that something like raw veggies or fruit such as an apple or a pear did the trick. Raw veggies and apples are crunchy and take time to chew, and they're not heavy in the sense of being calorie- or fat-dense, so chomping on those gave me something to do without overfilling me. This trick is particularly useful if you're the kind of person who snacks while preparing dinner. It's easy to sample so much before the meal that you're too full to eat it when it's ready. That's the time to break out the raw veggie snacks. They'll give your jaws something to do while not filling you up.

The purpose of this Action is learning to determine whether you need to eat for satisfaction or just for something to do. Sometimes you can just go for a walk, do a chore you've been putting off, change the pace of your current activity, or eat something that keeps your jaws busy.

Action #5: *Find the right balance*

Whole-wheat bread is a whole food, but it wouldn't be good if your diet consisted of 80 percent bread. Eggs are a whole food, but it wouldn't be good if your diet consisted of 80 percent eggs. Oranges are a whole food, but it wouldn't be good if your diet consisted of 80 percent oranges. Of course these examples are overstated. But they do underline an important consideration: an ideal diet isn't just about whole foods, it's also about variety and balance because the wrong balance will leave your body craving more food. The challenge is, how do you find that balance?

When I was in my dieting years I noticed that I had cravings for certain types of foods at different times. If I tried to follow the Atkins Diet and ate a big protein/fat-only breakfast (like eggs and bacon), within hours I craved carbs. If I tried a low-fat diet I found the opposite: I craved high-fat foods like bacon, cheese, or fried chicken. My body was very good at giving me metabolic messages; it was trying to tell me balance was important. Problem was, I wouldn't listen.

On the other hand, I also learned you can overdo the balance thing. Dr. Barry Sears' *Zone Diet*, which I also tried, is based on balancing every single meal and snack with a certain percentage of protein, carbs, and fat. While I understand the principle and the concept that balancing everything you eat is supposed to give you the optimal metabolic performance, I think it's overkill. Our bodies have evolved to handle variations within the food supply, and we don't need that level of micromanagement. Plus, after a while it gets really annoying.

The answer lies in learning to recognize the cravings you have and respond to them. I've emphasized that you should eat based on what you think you need. But you're not going to nail it every time. And your needs are going to change hour by hour and day by day because they'll be influenced by what you've eaten before and by your activity and stress levels. So you adjust.

Examples:

- If I feel the need for a high-protein breakfast and I eat a cheese omelet, come lunchtime, I'm done with the protein thing. All I want is some form of carbs: salad, vegetable soup, pasta, or something similar. So that's what I eat. And the next morning I won't want eggs, I'll want cereal.
- If I have bread for breakfast, I find I won't want a sandwich for lunch.
- If I have a salad for lunch, I won't want one for dinner—I may not even want one for a couple of days.
- If I have a big lunch, I'll want a light dinner.
- If I have a meal that's evenly balanced between protein, fat and carbs, I don't have any strong food preferences going into the next meal.

Over the course of a week it all works out. It's more important to balance your foods over the week or even over the month than meal by meal and snack by snack. And your body will tell you what it needs if you learn to listen.

Think of your foods in terms of categories: protein, carbs, and fats. For this Action, after you've eaten a meal that emphasizes one category of food, pay attention to what you seem to want over the next twenty-four hours. You'll probably have a taste for a different kind of food. It might not be a full-on craving, but it's a good bet you'll feel an inclination. If you have a big steak, maybe you won't want meat at your next meal. If you have spaghetti, you might not want more pasta or bread at your next meal. If you have a meal of fried foods you might want a less fatty meal next, such as a salad.

Track your taste informally off and on over a week or two. You'll likely see a pattern emerge and you can make a note of it in the workbook. If you listen, your body will communicate to you what it wants—so stay tuned for its feedback.

Action #6: Choose foods that satisfy

I've already talked about asking yourself what it is you really want as a basis of choosing your foods. But sometimes you need to consider the lasting power of what you select. I'm not a fan of the grazing method. If you like it and are comfortable with planning and carrying along enough snacks to keep you going, then that's fine. It doesn't work for me because:

- The more exposure I have to food, the more I eat.
- I don't want to have to be thinking about food all the time and lugging around a bunch of snacks.

With that in mind, I choose foods that have staying power. Typically, those are high in protein and have enough fat (animal or vegetable). You might think this means only meat, cheese, or eggs, but that's not so. Vegetarian fare will work just as well. A hearty bean soup with vegetables and whole-wheat pasta or brown rice, made with enough olive oil to give it substance, will do the trick. Oatmeal or other whole-grain cereal with butter or coconut oil, lots of nuts, and some fruit is good too. Or a whole-wheat cheese-and-tomato sandwich. It all comes down to what you like.

You should also choose foods you *enjoy*. If you plan meals you enjoy, you won't dread dinner at the end of the day—you'll look forward to it. And that anticipation will help you eat less *before* dinner. If you're going to have something you like, why spoil it by advance snacking? A little hunger can be a good thing. The important thing is to know what satisfies you based on the foods you enjoy.

For this Action, make a list of the whole foods you like that have this kind of staying power. Choose something from this list the next time you think it will be a long time between food availability.

RECALIBRATE YOUR PERCEPTIONS

The Context

What does perception have to do with it?

Perception is our view of the world. It may or may not be accurate, but it's what we see and feel and therefore it's what is real to us. It's the set of conclusions we've arrived at through our senses and a lifetime of experiences. We see and interpret everything through this set of conclusions. Perception is also about how we see ourselves relative to society's accepted norms. For example, if all your friends have giant-screen HDTVs and you can't afford one, you'll feel deprived. You might even go out and finance one even though you can't afford it. Unconsciously or not, we are constantly comparing ourselves to the norm and adjusting our perceptions and behavior accordingly.

So it is with our perceptions about food. From our senses, we learn what we like and dislike. But how much we should eat, what's good, what's not good, what we're supposed to eat, what we're not supposed to eat—we learn these from society's norms. Considering this country's obsession with quantity (more is always better), it should be no surprise that we learn to prefer cheap, convenient, processed foods because we can get more of them for our money. That's why, in my introduction to The Battle of Quantity, I said it's the most difficult battle of all. When quantity is the basis for the societal norm, all outside cues about eating reinforce that.

Consequently, all our quantity guidelines are *external, not internal*. We have no idea what amount of food is appropriate for us. We've never learned to associate a small amount of food with satisfaction. My dad had a phrase for it: "Your eyes are bigger than your stomach." There's a complete disconnect between the quantity we *think* is normal to eat and what it *should be*. We need to reset our perception so it's based on our own reality, not on what we've seen or learned in the past.

Some of the Actions ahead may seem trivial because they ask you to focus on how you think. But they are important because perception is a mental process and you need to know what your perception is to change it.

The objective

Recalibrating your Perceptions is a very important step in reactivating your built-in appestat. Your old perceptions obscure the signals your appestat is sending to you. As those perceptions disappear, the appestat signals come in stronger and faster. At first I could only tell if I'd eaten too much an hour after a meal or snack. After a while, though, the full signal started coming through midway through the meal.

Resetting your perceptions around quantity is one of the most difficult things to do, so be patient; if they're deep-rooted it will take time to displace them. During that time you can expect to fall back off and on. The Actions are tools you can apply whenever you find yourself struggling with finding and sticking to the right quantity for you. It takes practice to eat less. *You'll need to prove to yourself over and over that less is enough.* Once you truly feel it's enough at a physical level, the new perception becomes normal and consequently automatic.

Action #7: Eating without looking—the blindfold test

This first experiment is not for everyone. But it can give you a good feel for focusing on how your stomach feels without visual interference. One of the strongest cues that tell us how much to eat is visual presentation. The more food we see, the more we will likely eat, whether we're full or not. The blindfold test is just to get you started on tuning into what your stomach has to say.

Choose a meal or snack you commonly eat and *like*, that can be cut up into bite-sized pieces. For instance, try a peanut butter sandwich, boneless chicken, or cheese and crackers. Prepare the food, cut it up, and put a small amount on your plate. Then sit down at a table, put on a blindfold and eat the pieces slowly, taking a minute or so between bites. After each bite, notice how your stomach feels. If you finish what you put on your plate and you're still hungry, add some more. Stop when you think you've had enough, even it means leaving some pieces on the plate. Compare how much you ate with the blindfold on to how much you would have eaten without it. If you normally overeat, the amount you ate blindfolded will probably be less.

This Action is not something to do for every meal, but it's a good idea to try it a few times with different kinds of foods so you get more practice listening to your internal signals.

Action #8: Realign your association of quantity with satisfaction

"My cat eats more than that!"

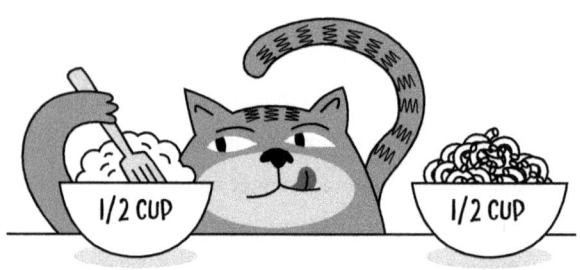

Another external signal we get is the so-called serving size, which is supposed to tell us how much is appropriate to eat at one time. But using this as a guide has a *real underlying dysfunction*: the implication that if we don't have a serving size reference (volume or weight), we'll have no idea how much to eat and when to stop. And unfortunately, because we've come to depend on said serving size, most of us don't know.

This condition is not a problem of gluttony, lack of will-power, or even habit. It is a problem of *perception*. What's happened is that we've developed a deep-rooted *visual association between quantity and satisfaction*. The only way to permanently fix this problem is to *destroy the old perception and replace it with a new one*.

I like to use a cat metaphor to illustrate our visual association with quantity. One day I took out a small custard cup and put a half cup of water in it. I did so because lots of food labels and diet recommendations specify a half cup as the serving size for cooked grains such as oatmeal, bulgur, and rice, as well as for cottage cheese, tuna salad, and pasta. Then I tried to imagine eating the same amount of some food I liked, and my immediate reaction was "Seriously?! My cat eats more than that! And it only weighs fifteen pounds!" The half-cup serving size seemed so ridiculously small, I couldn't believe that's all I should eat. But that's because I was using my eyes as a guide and not my stomach. Depending on my metabolic circumstances, one half cup might be enough or it might not.

The purpose of the next Action is to *begin* the process of destroying an old perception and replacing it with a new one. It's not a one-time Action; you'll need to repeat it often with various kinds of foods you like. But not all at once. As always: one change at a time. And after a few repetitions, it will become quite natural.

Starting with a meal or snack of your choice, measure out a half cup of something you like—egg salad, cottage cheese, tuna salad, mac and cheese, whatever—or make half a sandwich. Try not to think about what the quantity looks like compared to what you usually eat. Just eat it and wait a half hour. Evaluate your hunger level. If you feel full, write down the food and the quantity and add it to your this-is-enough-food list. If not, try it again a few more times. If it still leaves you feeling hungry, then maybe that serving size is too small for you. Increase it to three-quarters of a cup and try again. In either case, when you get to the point where you feel satisfied with a particular amount, make yourself picture that amount in your head as you think about your physical feeling of satisfaction.

The reason this is so important in *resetting normal* is that when you finally get it right, it puts you in the driver's seat. There's a world of difference between someone telling you that you can only eat a half cup of pasta and you *physically feeling* that a half cup of pasta is satisfying. With the former, you'll always be feeling deprived and wanting more; with the latter, you won't care.

And you'll stop thinking about how much your cat eats.

Action #9: Confront the perception of deprivation

Building on the cat metaphor: because we anticipate satisfaction visually, any amount that *looks* like less than we expect as "normal" generates a perception of deprivation. Subconsciously we think, "That doesn't look like enough," because we've become used to eating until we're stuffed. This line of thinking manifests itself as a resistance to eating less. It's why, the day before you go on a diet, you load up on everything you like. You might also find this a nagging problem when you eat at a restaurant: Should you order the small plate or the regular dinner? Just the *anticipation* of future deprivation is enough to set off stockpiling behavior. It's not a physiological reaction, it's a psychological one.

Confronting this perception takes experimentation. Take a minute or two to analyze your thinking when you're about to pack yourself a lunch or snack or when you're about to order at a restaurant, then again when you're done eating. What did your mind tell you about the quantity you *anticipated* would satisfy you vs. the quantity that actually did? If you went for the smaller quantity, did it satisfy you? If you went for the larger quantity, did you feel like you ate too much? Perhaps it made you think, "I knew I shouldn't have ordered that much." Then, the next time you encounter the same situation, instead of mindlessly going for the larger amount, modify your choice based on your earlier feedback.

Action #10 (optional): Employ the Power of One

One helping, that is.

The Power of One is another way to expose the fear of deprivation. This may not apply to everyone, but it applies to anyone who attacks a meal by taking multiple small helpings. It was an eye-opener for me and a critical turning point.

I came up with this idea while I was struggling to find ways to reduce the quantity I was eating. I'd tried the advice to use a smaller plate to make my portions appear larger, but I'd simply compensate by taking multiple small helpings. It finally occurred to me that by doing so, I never really knew how much I was eating and I thought it would be important to find out.

The experiment

My goal: Try to limit quantity by having only *one* plateful of food at dinner.

Day 1: To get myself over my initial resistance to the one-helping limit, I piled more food on my plate than I thought I could eat—kind of like many people do at all-you-can-eat restaurants. It looked like a humongous amount of food, and it was. It was so much I couldn't quite finish it all.

Day 2: I piled my plate full again, but not quite as high as on Day 1. It still looked like too much food, and again, it was. I finished it all, but an hour later I felt stuffed and wished I hadn't.

Day 3: I filled the plate again, reducing the amount more. It still looked like a lot of food. I finished it and felt a little stuffed, but not as much as I had the day before.

Day 4: I filled the plate again, reducing the quantity again. It still looked like a lot of food. I finished it but felt I was getting close to comfortable with the amount.

Day 5: I reduced the amount of food on the plate still more and finally felt just right. By this time, I had a pretty good idea how much I could put on my plate to fill me up yet prevent me from wanting second helpings. The interesting thing was that, compared to my usual small helpings, it still looked like too much food.

Day 6–12: I stuck with the one-helping plan, filling my plate with about the same amount as on Day 5, thinking it still looked to me like an awful lot of food, but eating it all anyway.

The surprising result

After two weeks of piling my plate full and eating it all, you'd think I would've gained weight even without taking second helpings of anything. But in fact, I lost weight. I don't know how much (my scale was in storage), but I knew I'd lost weight because my jeans were slightly loose around the waist.

This was a real wake-up call because what it told me was that *despite the seemingly large quantity of food I was eating, it was less than I'd been eating when I was taking multiple small helpings.* Sitting at the table and adding one spoonful of food to my plate at a time, *I'd had no idea how much food I'd been consuming.* Apparently, it had been a lot.

The revelation

This one-helping revelation was not only an eye-opener but a cause for celebration. Now I had a serious clue as to why I had so much trouble losing weight. With my small helpings I'd been deceiving myself. They made me *feel* like I wasn't eating much—it's just a spoonful, right? While in fact, I was *overeating.*

Now, if I told you it was easy to stick with this approach, I'd be lying. It wasn't. And it's because of the whole perception thing: even though I knew (intellectually) putting all that food on my plate would be plenty and satisfying, I had trouble enforcing the limit because psychologically, I just didn't like the idea of not having the option to take more. I was a lot like the whiny child who complains, "But I don't *want* to!" So it went in fits and starts. Sometimes I could stick to one helping, and sometimes I just didn't want to and slipped back into my old multiple-tiny-helpings habit. But overall, it did reduce the amount of food I ate, and my body size gradually started to shrink. Not a lot, but enough encourage me.

Long-term implications

You might be wondering how long I continued to try to apply The Power of One and if I still do. The answer to the first question is that I used it off and on for months, possibly a year (I don't remember exactly.) The answer to the second question is no. This experiment was a crucial turning point for me because it made me confront my quantity problem head on. However, once my appestat reactivation was complete, I no longer needed to use any superimposed tactics. I'm now on auto-pilot.

Some of us have a hard time resisting multiple helpings of food. That's why the small-plate recommendation doesn't always work: as I discovered, filling a small plate with multiple helpings only disguises the amount of food you consume. When you force yourself to stick with one plateful—even if it's a large plateful—you may find that you'll actually consume less than if you take more and more food, one spoonful at a time. If the multiple-helping syndrome applies to you, give the Power Of One a try.

Here's a guide:

Day 1: Estimate the amount of food you'll eat at your meal

Try to estimate the amount of food you're going to eat for a meal at home (where you could take multiple helpings). Put that amount on your plate and resist taking second or third helpings. For the first round, it's ok to err on the side of a lot of food.

Day 2: Adjust your estimate

If the plateful you took on Day 1 left you too full, put less on your plate this time. If you were still hungry after your one plateful, put more on your plate.

Days 3–7: Adjust your estimate each day

Based on the previous day's level of satisfaction with quantity, either increase or decrease the amount of food you dish on your single plateful.

Keep adjusting each day until you think you have it just right.

Days 8–12

If you still haven't hit the sweet spot, keep adjusting your quantity.

Evaluate

Did you find it easy or hard to stick to one helping? Do you feel lighter/thinner? Do you think you ate less by limiting yourself to one helping? If this exercise helped you get a better feel for how much you eat, continue to do it for several months and re-evaluate. At some point you probably won't need it anymore.

Action #11: Conquer portion envy

It seems to be part of the human mindset for us to compare ourselves to others. Am I as smart? Am I thinner or fatter? Am I richer or poorer? Can you eat more than I can? We have a *perception* that if the universe were truly fair, these disparities wouldn't exist.

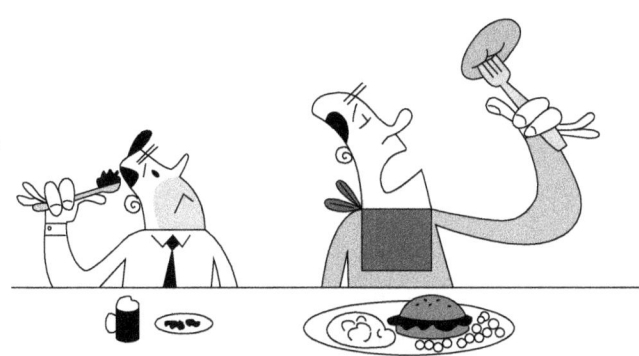

When it comes to food comparisons, it starts early. "He got more than me!" or "Can I have more than her?" are common complaints from children. And it seems we don't altogether outgrow that thinking. I call this "portion envy" because those of us who enjoy eating always wish we could eat more. Naturally, we're envious of the people who can do so without apparent consequences: we'd like to be able to eat as much as that guy over there can. This is completely unrealistic, of course, because we're all different. If you're six feet tall, you need more food than someone who is five feet tall. If you're muscular, you need more food than someone who is not. If you have a job that requires a lot of physical exertion, you need more food than someone whose job is working at a computer.

Sometimes it's a matter of metabolism. Or age. Or a combination of any of the above attributes. I remember one time when I was in my early fifties and I had lunch with a couple of female acquaintances in their early thirties. They each scarfed down large burgers, fries, and a beer while I ate broiled fish and left my fries on my plate. They were both thin and I was not. Not fair! My husband is six feet tall so it's natural for him to consume a lot more food than I can. Not fair!

Today, as I sit writing this, I'm at a stage where just about everyone can eat more than I can. At about five feet two and in my seventies, my true food needs are pretty small. Over time I've come to terms with that. But it wasn't easy. I had to stop associating my enjoyment of food with quantity and *re-associate it with quality.* I had to get used to the idea that if I eat slowly and appreciate the quality of what I'm eating, that's a much more rewarding experience than scarfing down a ton of food and feeling like a blimp afterward. I can enjoy my smaller meal just as much as the person across from me eating twice as much.

It takes mental practice to stop comparing yourself to others. When you've done the Actions for recalibrating your perceptions, you'll have a solid foundation for resisting portion envy. This Action builds on the concept of focusing inward rather than outward. Stop looking at how much everyone else is eating. Instead, associate the amount of food on your own plate with how your stomach feels—particularly with your level of satisfaction. Remind yourself that eating is not a contest. If you feel satisfied with what you ate, why should you care how much anyone else ate?

Action #12: Change your perceptions as you get older

I hear a lot about both women and men gaining weight after they pass a "certain age." With women it's typically blamed on hormonal changes. I haven't heard much speculation about why it happens with men. However, once again I'm going to propose my own theory based on my experience. I won't argue that hormones have no effect—they do. But I have a slightly different twist on what causes us to gain weight at a certain time of life.

My theory is that as we get older, a change in hormone balance slows down our metabolism. We can't be as active as we could when we were in our twenties. We don't need energy for baby production and child-raising. In general, we slip into a more reflective, supportive mode rather than a set-the-world-on-fire mode. Since we don't need the level of energy we used, to we also don't need the same quantity of food we used to eat.

But here's the rub: if we haven't changed our perception about how much we can eat in this new stage of life—if we're still thinking about how much we *used* to be able to eat and relying on our *visual* evaluation of portion size—we'll continue to eat the amount we used to and consequently we'll gain weight. You might call it a special case of portion envy, except that in this case you're envious of your former self instead of someone else.

You don't have to fix this problem by taking corrective hormones. You can fix it by changing your perception of how much food is appropriate for you. And you do that by learning to listen to your satisfaction signals instead of visual cues. You need to get your perception in line with reality. This is true whether you're male or female.

When I look at the food that satisfies me today, it seems pitifully small compared to what I used to eat. But destroying my old perceptions and replacing them with more appropriate ones has allowed me to become comfortable with it. It's now my normal. I, too, started gaining weight around menopause. But once I reset my normal I had no trouble stopping the weight gain and getting down to where I needed to be. I no longer perceive smaller portions as a deprivation. It's just the amount I normally eat.

If you're in this stage of life, pay special attention at every meal to how much (or little) it takes to actually fill you up. Think about what you used to eat and ask yourself the following: Do you really need as much food as you used to? Or are you eating those same portions out of habit? As with fighting portion envy, focus inward on your level of satisfaction rather than the external visual of what's on your plate or your memory of what you used to eat.

Action #13: Destroy and replace one old perception

Finally, I come to the heart of the matter. This is where the real change happens. It's in this process that you finally jettison external portion control as the solution to losing weight and set your internal portion control on auto-pilot. It takes a little persistence and patience, but it's well worth the effort. Once it's done, you *never* have to worry about portion control again.

To destroy and replace old perceptions, you apply the techniques you learned in the Goldilocks Quest, and exploring your perceptions around each of your problematic snacks and meals in turn. Here's an example of how I did it.

I started with my Saturday breakfast because it was a predictable ritual. Saturday morning breakfast meant fresh-squeezed orange juice, eggs, bacon, toast, jam, and coffee. The only thing that varied was the way I prepared the eggs.

For most of my life, a breakfast like that consisted of two eggs, two or three pieces of bacon, and sometimes two pieces of toast. But I began to notice that eating this amount—even though it seemed normal to me—made me feel too full (the one-hour feedback loop). So I started experimenting.

The first week of my experiment I decided to cut back to one egg, one piece of bacon, and one piece of toast. First time around that went fine. I felt good an hour later, so you'd think that would be the end of it. But no. That was just the beginning.

I had good intentions of having the smaller quantity the next Saturday. But I woke up hungry and when it was time to decide how many eggs and bacon I should cook, I decided I needed two eggs. Why? Because one egg doesn't look like much on a plate. Especially if it's a boiled egg. (It looks like: "My cat eats more than that!") So I drifted back to my two-of-everything mode. Of course, an hour later I felt like I'd swallowed a bowling ball—I was way too full. I made a note to myself: next Saturday back to one of everything.

And I did that: the following week I had one of everything and I felt good. Great. Had I fixed myself? No. What followed was weeks of a back-and-forth waltz between one egg and two. Intellectually I knew one egg was enough, but my perception of normal kept nagging me that one egg was so small, it meant deprivation. I asked myself over and over, "You *know* one is enough—what's so hard about just eating *one*?" What was hard was just *thinking* about limiting myself to one because in my mind one wasn't normal. Everyone else seemed to be able to eat two.

So how did I finally win this battle? I won it with persistence. I made it a point to evaluate how I felt after breakfast every Saturday. And I kept associating how I felt after eating one egg with good and how I felt after eating two with bad. As time went on the number of times I opted for one increased and the number of times I opted for two decreased because I could recall that association before I made the decision. Finally, one egg, one bacon, and one piece of toast became my new normal. I'd destroyed my old two-egg perception and I was done. Since then, it's never been a question I ask myself. It doesn't matter how many eggs other people around me are eating, or what it looks like, one is normal for me.

The goal of this exercise is to destroy your old perception of a normal quantity and replace it with one that's appropriate for you at this time in your life. Once you've done this, you'll have your own built-in portion-control mechanism and you won't have to impose an artificial one. You won't have to apply this process to every single meal you have. Your success might be slow at first, but once you get the feel of it, it should go much faster.

Here is a guide on how to do this:

Prepare:

1) Choose a meal or snack you eat regularly and tend to overeat.
2) Through experimentation, find the quantity of food that feels just right—one that passes the one-hour-later feedback test.
3) Set that quantity as your new normal-quantity goal.

Then practice:

1) Each time you're going to eat that meal or snack, try to imagine how you felt when you ate the just-right quantity and how you felt when you ate too much.
2) Try to convince yourself to choose the just-right quantity.
3) Eat according to whatever your decision was.

4) Note how you feel one hour later.
5) Go back to #1.

Practice until you're so comfortable with your new perception that making the right decision is no longer a struggle.

As your new perception begins to take hold, there may be times when you choose the larger quantity but then don't feel like you can finish it comfortably. That's a good thing. Don't be afraid to leave food on your plate. Try not to serve yourself more than you can eat, but if you do, practice leaving it there. It's not going to feed starving children, and eventually you'll be able to serve yourself the right amount.

Action #14: Continue to destroy and replace perceptions, one at a time

Once you have that first new perception in line, choose another meal or snack where you typically overeat. Apply the process in Action #13 to destroy and replace your usual quantity with a more comfortable amount. Get that one in line and tackle another one. Repeat ... until you rarely overeat. You'll probably never get to choosing just the right amount 100 percent of the time, but you don't have to. Just fixing your perceptions most of the time will make a huge difference.

MANAGING THE SOCIAL CONTEXT

The Context

As if it weren't bad enough that we have to battle our own perceptions and deceptions about how much we should eat, we have to deal with the perceptions of others and with social customs. How do you survive in a world where everyone else is eating themselves to death and expects you to do the same?

The social implications of eating less. When we reduce the amount we eat, that creates an activity void. For instance, it's now normal for me to eat small meals, which may not take much time. But I still have a need to socialize while eating, whether it's a family dinner, a business lunch, or a couple of friends having coffee—it's just part of what it means to be human. Therein lies the problem: if I'm finished eating in a few minutes, how do I stretch out the socialization? After much experimentation, I finally figured out some techniques to deal with this situation.

Action #15: Note the time required to eat whole foods vs. processed foods

One way to take longer to eat less is to eat whole foods. You probably realized this after you started replacing the processed foods in your diet with whole ones.

I mentioned earlier that one of the advantages of whole foods is that their natural package is part of their value; an apple, for instance, has more nutritional value than apple juice. But because of that, you actually have to chew these foods before you swallow them. You can swallow a donut in one or two minutes, but if you have a large salad it's going to take some time to dispose of. You can drink a glass of orange juice in a minute, but if you eat the whole orange it may take ten or fifteen minutes. You can throw down a chicken nugget in one bite—it's mostly chicken mush—but you'll have to work a little harder on a piece of grilled chicken.

You might think this is a no-brainer, but to experience it for yourself, set aside a little time to make a comparison. Pick a processed food you usually eat and a similar whole food. For example, orange juice vs. a whole orange; a donut vs. a slice of artisan whole-wheat toast; a half cup of raw carrots vs. a half cup of potato chips. Time yourself. Note how long it takes to eat the processed food compared to the whole food.

Action #16: S-l-o-w down

Another way to take longer to eat less is to slow down. I've talked to people who eat very fast—I call them NASCAR eaters—and they tell me that eating slowly is difficult for them. I'm not sure if it's because they just have so much to do that they're always in a hurry, or they wait until they're so hungry they feel like they need to wolf down their food, or it's just habit. But slowing down to eat is very important because:

- Digestion starts in your mouth—food mixes with your saliva and that starts the breakdown process, giving your stomach a head start.
- It gives your built-in appestat time to measure your satisfaction level.
- It prevents you from dumping too much into your stomach at once before you can even sense if you're full.
- Eating should be enjoyable—you should eat slowly enough that you can actually taste what you're eating.

If you're a NASCAR eater, you probably finish before anyone else at the table. If you eat at turtle speed, you're probably the last to finish. Or you might be somewhere in between.

Test yourself the next time you eat with others: which one are you? If you eat too fast, make a conscious effort to chew a little longer, take a breath between bites (count silently to ten or twenty), take smaller bites, chat with your colleagues, or do anything else you can think of to slow yourself down. It's also important to slow down when drinking sodas or alcoholic beverages. If you find yourself guzzling your drinks, try to make yourself sip them instead.

Action #17: Resist evangelizing

People aren't always open to new ideas or ideas they'd prefer to ignore. They may be offended if you change your eating habits then start lecturing them about what you think they should do. For me, the secret to managing my journey was not making a big deal about it. I chose not to evangelize the changes I was making unless someone asked me about it—and then I kept it short and cryptic. I respected others' eating habits but quietly maintained my own. Anyone who hadn't known me when I was overweight just assumed I never was and I'd always eaten the same way I ate that day.

When you are in a social situation, resist the urge to lecture. You can be a mild evangelist for *Resetting Normal* if someone asks you about it. Otherwise, the less said, the better. Chances are, no one will notice you eat less or differently and it won't become a point of discussion.

Learn to handle other people's perceptions of a normal quantity

We can change our own perception around quantity, but we have no control over anyone else's. If we reset our normal quantity to something smaller than the societal normal, we're out of sync with everyone else and eventually they're going to notice. We need to find ways to deal with this politely.

Action #18: Be a quantity-conscious guest

According to the typical quantity perception, people expect you to eat a lot. If you eat out with others and you don't, people think you don't like their food. You might even offend them if you don't ask for a second helping. I used to be one of those people. That has changed since I reset normal; I no longer look at quantity consumption as proof of approval. I can love a particular food yet be quite happy eating a small portion, and I'm ok with giving others the space to eat as much or little as they like. However, society at large isn't there yet.

For example, sometimes pressure comes in the form of "You have to have some—I made it especially for you." Or "It's your birthday—you can have this [gigantic] piece of cake." Or "It's Thanksgiving—everyone overeats." People usually mean well, but their perceptions and expectations can get the better of them. Perhaps you know some people like that. There are ways to work around them politely;

they are, after all, just trying to make you feel good. However, be careful that you aren't one of them yourself.

You can be just as appreciative if you eat less or have switched to different foods, but you need to find a polite way to communicate that to your host. Don't become so obnoxious and self-righteous about your changes that you alienate your friends. Nature, wisely, thrives on diversity—it's only human society that wants everyone to be the same. So respect everyone's choices, even if you don't agree with them.

The next time you're a guest there are four ways you can protect your dietary decisions without insulting your host:

- If you know ahead of time what the menu is and there's nothing on it that suits you, bring something you like and present it as a polite contribution.
- Eat slowly and people probably won't notice you're eating less.
- If you can serve yourself, take very small helpings at first, then make sure they notice you go back for seconds.
- If the host keeps encouraging you to eat more than you want, try responding with something like, "This is really wonderful! I love the [whatever] that you put into it. I'm just really full—I can't eat as much as I used to."

Action #19: Be a quantity-conscious host

When you're the host, it's important to understand that your guests may not have the same quantity requirements as you, so be flexible in a respectful way. Provide plenty of food for those who want it but don't force it on others—give your guests choices.

- If you're pre-loading the plates, don't overload them. Put extra on the table so your guests can take more if they want.
- Make your guests feel comfortable asking for more but don't pressure them.
- Don't say things that would make your guests feel guilty about either gorging or not gorging themselves.

Action #20: Manage the social implications of our Western lifestyle

Lack of time to eat at work is one of the downsides of our Western lifestyle. Lots of work places allow just a half hour for lunch—that's their *perception* of how long lunch should take. If you're trying to eat whole foods for lunch, finishing in a half hour can be difficult. This leaves you with two bad choices: 1) eat processed foods you can force down in that half hour, or 2) eat whole foods but do so at your desk, where you can take your time. Neither is optimal, but of the two, the second one is better.

Even more problematic than that, however, is that some jobs require lots of meetings. I've observed colleagues having so many, they're scheduled back-to-back with zero time for lunch. And in those meetings, whole foods are a problem. Many—like a salad, an apple, or even nuts—are noisy. Which wouldn't be a problem if everyone else was eating something like that. But if you're the only one, it's embarrassing. It's also uncomfortable if everyone else finishes their processed-food lunch in fifteen minutes and you're still munching away beyond a half hour. Most people in this situation cave in and just bring candy or a food bar or hit the vending machine in a five-minute break, and that's not good on a regular basis.

Unfortunately, there aren't many good solutions to this dilemma. However, there are a number of packaged soups on the market today that are made with whole foods—lentil- or bean-based—and only require microwave heating. (As always, double-check the label for additives.) One of these, plus some hummus and crackers, or half a peanut butter sandwich on whole-grain bread, or cut-up chicken or something similar, and you have a whole-foods lunch that isn't noisy and probably won't take too long to consume. The good news is that there's a growing interest in these types of food products so new ones frequently appear in the market.

Another challenge is to avoid the all-too-many sweet snacks many of us find lying around the workplace. You can compensate for this phenomenon by going on the offensive: if your colleagues are bringing in donuts, cookies, and other similar snacks, when it's your turn, bring in some artisan bread, butter, cream cheese, a few other cheeses, and grapes. You'll be surprised how pleased they'll be.

BUILD A DEFENSE AGAINST OUTSIDE INFLUENCES
The Context
To reinvigorate your own appestat, bolster your defenses against the influence of experts and the food industry. You can resist both of them with some simple techniques that help you change your mindset, listen to your own body's feedback, and watch out for yourself. Since we live with a system that bombards us with what-to-dos, rewards us for buying more, and punishes us for buying less, it's up to us to stay aware and avoid the pressure as much as possible.

Action #21: Choose quality over quantity

Always choose quality over quantity—go for the quality product and you'll eat less in the long run. Buy satisfying products and enjoy them for what they are. Don't choose products based solely on their calorie values. It does you absolutely no good to eat a low-calorie food if you'll be hungry a half hour later. Choose products based on their whole-food nutritional values, what you think you need to eat, and the level of satisfaction they provide.

If you've worked your way through the Actions this far, you should already be good at this, but because there's so much pressure these days to focus on calories, continue to practice it regularly as part of your defense arsenal.

Action #22: Manage snacktivity

The food industry has fostered a demand for frequent snacking, developing products specifically designed for this purpose, marketing them heavily, and making them available everywhere. Potato chips, pretzels, food bars, and hundreds of variations on those themes are in our faces 24/7, encouraging us to engage in what I call *snacktivity*—continual snacking activity.

It's easy to get caught up in snacktivity when you're heavily dependent on processed foods because they never fill you up for very long. The primary defense against snacktivity is choosing quality foods that satisfy. When you're full, you're much less likely to snack. Caveat: if you have a long-time habit of snacking—even if you've replaced most of your processed foods—put snack foods out of sight for a while to keep you from mindlessly attacking them.

Once you've completely reset normal this deception won't be necessary. I have a bar in the family room and on the counter I keep containers of pretzels, Cheezits, cashews, chocolate candy, or other snack items, because every once in a while I want some. But I don't eat them all the time just because they're there. I always apply the principle of asking myself what I really want before I eat—and those snacks may sit there for weeks at a time, untouched.

Action #23: Resist food-industry deals

Be selective. One of the secrets to conquering our tendency to eat more than we need, especially of processed foods, is to limit how much we buy. If it's not in the house you can't eat it. It's *normal* in our society to look for these deals and grab them whenever we can. To reset your normal buying habits, don't focus on the potential savings of the deal. Focus instead on what you and your family *actually* need and what you'll gain by resisting the deal. You'll spend less money in the long run and you'll eat less food. The temptation to overbuy is not trivial; it takes practice and persistence to change your mindset and reset normal.

The next time you're confronted by a deal that tempts you to buy more than usual, stop and ask yourself the following:
- What quantity would I normally buy?
- Is this something that I (and my family) *should* eat more of?
- Is it perishable?
- How much more will I actually spend if I take the deal?

Then make your decision based on the best purchase for the situation.

Action #24: Resist restaurant pressure

Most of the major chain restaurants employ a bevy of researchers to design their menu items. These researchers try to figure out the optimal amount of fat, salt, sugar to make you crave them and consequently eat too much. This has been well documented in *The End of Overeating*[18].

Two-egg breakfasts used to be the norm. Now it's three, four or even five eggs. Add cheese and ham, sausage or bacon, hash brown potatoes, and two pieces of toast and that's a huge amount of food. Sandwiches and salads for lunch can be gigantic. If you order a pasta dish, it's likely to be made with at least a half pound of pasta. Coffee shops, for the most part, only serve super-size bagels, muffins, and pastries—all three times the size of what normal used to be thirty years ago.

Pizza shops use the same more-for-your-money strategy as the supermarkets. They usually offer the extra-large size at what seems a considerable discount. If you only want a small pizza, you're going to pay more. They also use the low/non strategy I described in the section on beating the Marketing Machine. One commercial for Papa Murphy's Pizza (6/2014) pushed a pizza with "25 percent less fat" and "35 percent fewer calories," finishing the pitch with, "Go ahead, take another slice." They're not trying to help you consume less fat and fewer calories; they're trying to sell you more pizza.

The best way to resist this pressure is to continue to practice ignoring the physical quantity of food. Instead, focus inward and evaluate your satisfaction as you eat. The operative word here is *enjoy*. Don't rush through your meal, and remember that if you get full you can always ask for a doggie bag.

The next time you're out eating and you're confronted with the restaurant quantity problem, try to apply one or more of the following suggestions:
- Focus on enjoying the quality of the food, not the quantity.
- If you know you're going to eat dinner out at a nice place, refrain from eating much during the day so you can actually consume more quantity later without overstuffing.
- If it's too much food for you, steel yourself to the idea of a doggie bag or just leave the food on your plate—it gets easier with practice.
- Avoid all-you-can-eat restaurants.
- For buy-more deals (like pizza), apply the anti-buy-more tactics in "Resist food-industry deals."
- Learn to apply the feedback loop so you can tell when you've had enough. Then just stop eating, no matter what. If there's ice cream left over in the dish, so what? If you only eat half that bagel or pastry, so what? The world is not going to end. And you can always eat more tomorrow if you want.

MANAGING HOLIDAYS, VACATIONS, AND BUSINESS TRAVEL
The Context

Eating too much on holidays and vacations is as traditional and American as apple pie. The typical cycle is overindulgence followed by regret followed by dieting. But it doesn't have to be this way. I can't deny there are some trouble spots you need to deal with when traveling and celebrating, but there are solutions. Reset normal and it will never be an issue for you again.

For one thing, you have some protection from the strange effect of short-term overeating. Surprisingly, I've observed that the body has a different way of dealing with short-term overeating than long-term. I don't have a scientific explanation for this phenomenon, so I'll explain using metaphors.

How homeostasis helps us

You don't have to optimize your metabolism minute by minute and day by day because your body is capable of managing much longer cycles. It doesn't require the same nutritional elements in the same quantities every single day. Weekly, monthly, and seasonal adjustments are perfectly within its control. And why would we think otherwise? From the earliest times, our food supply has varied by the seasons. Fruits and other edible plants were available in the summer and fall but not in winter.

Protein sources were seasonal as well, depending on an animal's life cycle. Through technology, we now have all foods available to us all year long, but our bodies can still deal with short-term deficits and surpluses like those we experience with holidays and vacations.

I think there are two states your body keeps track of: what is normal and what is not normal. When it encounters something it thinks is not normal, a process called homeostasis kicks in. This is the process your body uses to try to keep everything on an even keel. Your body is used to you at a certain weight and wants to keep it there. If you eat too little, it may slow down your metabolism to keep you from losing weight—this is one reason why dieting can be so difficult. On the other hand, if you eat too much, it does something else to keep you from gaining.

Soft weight vs. hard weight

What is that something else? Well, I don't know exactly, but I describe it as follows:

Your metabolism detects what I call soft weight and hard weight. What I've observed is that if I overeat for up to ten days—maybe two weeks at the outside—the excess food seems to go into a kind of temporary storage. When I stop overeating, this excess soft weight slips away easily. All I need to do is return to my normal consumption, and within a week the extra weight disappears by itself. But the cutoff point is somewhere between ten days and two weeks. If I overeat for more than two weeks, that excess food goes into long-term storage as hard weight, and then it's hard to get rid of.

Imagine your metabolic processes having the following conversation for the first ten days:

Stomach: Watch out—here comes a boatload of food.

Bloodstream monitor: Whoa, that *is* a lot of stuff. Hey Pancreas and Kidneys—what are we gonna do with all this?

Pancreas and Kidneys: I don't know—it's definitely more than we're used to. But let's hold onto it where we can get to it easily. It's probably a temporary windfall and we might need it—who knows what this body's going to do next? Might run a marathon for all we know, and if we convert it to fat and store it away, we'll just have to go get it and convert it back again. And we don't get overtime for that.

Now imagine your metabolic processes having the following conversation *after* ten days:

Stomach: It's still coming in—tons of it.

Bloodstream monitor: Ok. Hey Pancreas and Kidneys—this stuff is still flooding in. Time we had a conversation about what to do now.

Pancreas and Kidneys: Well, we're running out of temporary storage here. Looks like this is going to be the new normal, so let's just start converting it to fat and storing it away.

Another way to look at is to think of soft weight like a money-market account: you get a little less interest, but you can get to it easily if you need it. Opposite that you can think of hard weight like a thirty-year Treasury bond: it's there for the long term in a place that's not easily accessible.

Every year over the Thanksgiving holiday I eat my share of turkey, mashed potatoes, gravy, stuffing, and pie, but I don't try to cram it all into one day. Instead, I eat some every day over the long weekend. That includes potatoes, gravy, pie and all, Thursday through Sunday. The important qualifier in this situation is that I don't stuff myself every single day—I eat my own normal portions. But I get to spread the enjoyment over four days. Come Monday, I'm done. By that time, I've had my fill and I'm happy to go back to my normal eating habits. And I have no permanent weight gain.

I have absolutely no idea what the scientific explanation for this phenomenon is, but I do know that it happens to me the way I described. I can replicate it every time I have eaten more than usual for a short period of time. The important takeaway from this observation is that the cutoff point is between ten days and two weeks. If your overeating window is less than that, you don't need to worry. If it's longer than that, you need to employ the strategies described earlier for reducing overall quantity.

Outside of not worrying about short-term results, here are some Actions you can take to help you manage holidays, vacations, and business trips.

Action #25: Tolerate a little hunger

If it's a holiday or you're on vacation, avoid eating constantly. Don't eat like every meal is your last. Instead, choose where and what you want to eat most, let yourself build up anticipation for it, and enjoy those times without guilt.

If you're on business travel, you might be more limited in your choices about what, where, and when you can eat. Experiment with ways to eat less at unimportant functions and reserve your appetite for the important ones.

Action #26: Select your foods carefully

Where possible, choose quality, satisfying foods and enjoy them slowly.

Action #27: Keep as active as you can

Refer to the section on supercharging your everyday activity for suggestions on how to keep your body in motion, especially if you're on a business trip. If it's a holiday, help with the preparations. If you're on vacation, get plenty of rest, but in between choose activities that keep you on the move (walking is always great for this). And these days most hotels have mini-gyms, so take advantage of this if there are no other options.

Action #28: Enjoy yourself

You don't have to be fanatical or guilt-ridden for taking time off. Keep in mind the soft weight vs. hard weight phenomenon. Try not to stuff yourself and sit the whole time, but otherwise enjoy this break in your routine. As long as it doesn't last for more than two weeks, it will be easy to return to normal.

Action #29: Return to your new normal

Don't stress about holidays and vacations. As best as you can, try to eat according to your new normal and don't worry about the rest. And don't worry about potential weight gain. If you were to get on the scale the morning after holidays or vacations, you would undoubtedly see a rise in your weight. After your holiday/vacation/business trip, DO NOT GET ON THE SCALE AND DO NOT THINK ABOUT GOING ON A DIET! Simply return to your new normal eating and activity routines, and within a few weeks whatever temporary weight you gained will disappear by itself.

The idea that eating right during the holidays requires discipline and determination encapsulates what is wrong with the current dietary approach. Once you've reset normal, this is simply *not true*. I don't have to exert any discipline or determination anymore. Holiday and vacation eating is something I look forward to without fear. I enter January pretty close to the way I entered November. And I invite you to think about that.

Measuring Success

The Battle of Quantity is definitely the most difficult because you have to overcome others' perceptions as well as your own. You may not have to do all the Actions to succeed; choose the ones that fit you best. Don't try to do them all at once, but be prepared to do some over and over—that's the only way to destroy your old perceptions and replace them with new ones. Of all the suggestions, I think the most important one is the Goldilocks Quest, because learning to recognize your satisfaction point is the foundation of restoring your built-in appestat.

Success: You've won the Battle of Quantity when:

- You ignore outside signals about how much to eat and focus solely on your internal satisfaction level.
- You rarely, if ever feel stuffed, or too full at night to comfortably fall asleep.
- You aren't constantly hungry, thinking about food all the time.
- You don't cave in to pressure to eat more than you want.
- You can gracefully manage guest/host situations around quantity.
- You enjoy vacation and holiday eating but don't use them as an excuse to stuff yourself into oblivion.
- You don't end your vacations and holidays with thoughts about dieting.

NOTES

CHAPTER 11
THE FINAL FRONTIER

The Context

Many of you have been waiting to hear this part. Perhaps it's your main goal, and you're wondering why this section is way at the end and takes up only a fraction of this book. But the reason is simple: once you've won all the other battles, losing weight is trivial.

The Last Challenge

LOSING WEIGHT

Action #1: Status check

The state of body and mind is important because you can't start losing weight until you've stopped gaining it. By this time, you should have a baseline—a new normal. And now all you need to do is tweak your quantity just a little bit more. When you've won The Battle of the Mind, The Battle of Activity, The Battle of Quality, and all of The Battle of Quantity you should have the following strengths that you didn't have before:

- You have weight stability.
- You are off the yo-yo diet cycle—no more binges and recriminations.
- You look for ways to be active—you are no longer a couch potato.
- You eat mostly quality foods you enjoy.
- You feel satisfied with what you eat.
- You don't have extreme food cravings anymore.
- You can tolerate a little hunger now and then.

When this represents your current normal, you may already have lost weight, but if not, you're ready to start.

Action #2: Understand the process

Three rules:

1) Do not weigh.
2) Do not decide on a size goal.
3) Do not try to rush your progress.

The first rule is obvious—and you should have given up the scale in the Battle of the Mind. The second one is a variation on the first: tracking success according to size will put you right back into a diet mentality.

The third rule requires a little more explanation. The reason you shouldn't try to rush your progress has to do with your metabolism. Remember earlier when I described homeostasis? Your body tries to maintain stability by keeping you at the same weight it recognizes as normal. If you reduce your food intake drastically, your metabolism will react, slowing down and tempting you to eat more by sending you hunger signals. Some experts advise that to counter this state, you have to shock your body even more by ramping up your activity or even reducing your intake further—basically *forcing it* to accept the different normal. This is unpleasant, to say the least, and not always successful.

I have another way—a sneaky one. I've found that if I reduce my food intake very slightly and adjust the proportions of certain foods, I can actually trick my body into thinking things are just the same as they've always been. And a little at a time, I will lose weight without any drastic kickback from my metabolism.

When and how to cut back. Your choice for this is personal. The goal is to cut back on the amount of food you eat just two or three days a week. Which meal you choose for that depends on your own eating schedule and preferences.

I chose to cut back on dinner twice a week because, being a morning person, I tend to go to bed early, and if I'm asleep, I won't notice any hunger. Since I happen to like soup, I chose to have a bowl of soup—not just broth but something substantial like chicken vegetable with noodles. It was enough to fill me up because of the liquid content, but still lighter than a regular meat/vegetables/potatoes dinner. I did not give up my evening glass of wine, by the way.

So for me, twice a week, dinner was a glass of wine and a bowl of soup. And that was all it took to gradually nudge the weight downward. *You see, once your eating habits are stable, small tweaks make a difference.* It's not the same as some health expert calculating that if you drink one less soda a day, in a year you will lose [xx] pounds. The principle is the same: reducing calories over the long term will cause you to lose weight. But metabolism being what it is, you can never guarantee the loss of a specific number of pounds. And it only works if you haven't compensated somewhere else. If you drink one less soda per day but have a triple venti mocha latte or eat a couple of cookies instead, it's not going to get you anywhere. To lose weight by small reductions, you *must* have a relatively stable diet to begin with.

Action #3: Decide when to lighten up

Now that you understand how it works, choose two or three mealtimes a week when you think you'd feel ok with eating less. They should be on different days of the week, not consecutive. They could be different meals (lunch one day, dinner the next), but it's probably easier to make them the same.

The primary criterion is that each one should come at a time when you can tolerate a little extra hunger. You don't want to get to a point where you feel starving, because if you do your metabolism will fight back.

This should be a personal decision, but here are a few possibilities:
- If you go to bed early, choose dinner because you'll be asleep before you notice anything different.
- If you always have a bedtime snack, choose that.
- If you normally eat a big lunch, that might be a good choice.

Everyone's schedule and tolerances are different, so the answer is individual. Just pick two meals for a starting point. If it turns out that they aren't optimal, you can always switch to something different later.

Action #4: Decide how to lighten up

There are two rules for this:
1) Keep it simple. If you have to go through a lot of extra preparation, you'll get tired of it and quit.
2) Make sure your light meal is *something you like and enjoy*. You should be able to look forward to this meal just as much as any other meal—it should *never* feel like a punishment.

There are multiple possibilities for this, but here are a few suggestions:
- Cut what you would normally eat by about a third.
- Prepare something entirely different, such as a soup and/or salad—but make sure it's not so wimpy you'll be starving a half hour later.
- Substitute a double green vegetable portion in place of carbs like pasta, rice, bread or potatoes.
- Double your protein item and skip the dense (potatoes, pasta, rice, etc.) carbs altogether.
- Have a little fruit for dessert.

Action #5: Just do it

Start your planned changes and keep doing it for at least one month. If you find some psychological or physical resistance, remind yourself: these lighter meals are only two or three times per week, so you're not on a long-term deprivation schedule. You can always look forward to your normal meals the next day. Or perhaps you need to change which meals you should lighten up. Remind yourself it's not forever.

Remain open to serendipity. If you find that you're not really that hungry at one of your regular meals, or you work through your normal lunch and find you could comfortably wait until dinner, take advantage of that to eat less. Always be mindful of the primary *Resetting Normal* principle: only eat when you're hungry.

Action #6 (optional): Adjust quantity based on food types

If you've lightened your meals for a month and don't feel like you're making any progress, you might need to adjust the balance of your meals and snacks by choosing different food types. When I was growing up in the 1950s, foods were generally divided this way:

Type of food	Examples
Protein	Red meat, pork, chicken, fish, eggs, cheese
Non-starchy vegetables	Lighter vegetables, such as lettuce, asparagus, broccoli, cauliflower, cucumber, onions, tomatoes
Starchy vegetables	Denser vegetables such as potatoes, corn, peas, pumpkin, winter squash, dried beans
Starch	Grains, noodles, rice
Bread	Any type
Fruit	Fresh or canned
Dessert	Cakes, cookies, pies, etc.

With these classifications, a balanced meal plan was easy. All you needed was one of each of the following:

- One protein
- One non-starchy vegetable
- One starch or starchy vegetable
- One fruit or dessert
- Bread (optional, but usually served)

I still use this as a guideline today with the exception that since bread is a starch, I don't serve it with other starches. You may be accustomed to having garlic bread with spaghetti and meat sauce, but bread and spaghetti double the starch content, so nix that. Here are some menu samples of how to apply this approach.

Protein	Non-starchy veggie	Starch or starchy veggie	Fruit or Dessert
Chicken	Broccoli	Butternut squash	Strawberries
Meatballs	Salad	Spaghetti	Grapes
Fish	Spinach	Rice pilaf	Vanilla pudding
Cheese omelet	Asparagus	Bread	Pears
Beef stew	String beans	Potatoes	Apple pie

[Note: This approach would need to be modified for vegetarian menus since those sources of protein are plant-based, but the principle is the same.]

What does this balance have to do with losing weight? Some of us are very sensitive to carbohydrates like bread, pasta and potatoes, even when the grains are whole. If you're like that (I am), your Action here is to reduce the dense carbs, replacing some of them with a bigger portion of green vegetables (salad, broccoli, string beans, etc.) and your protein source. Don't eliminate those carbs altogether because that will only trigger cravings, just throttle back a little bit.

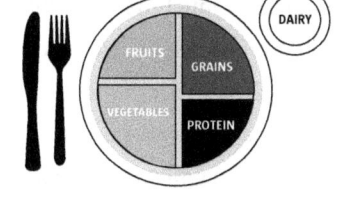

The latest USDA "food pyramid" (which is no longer a pyramid but is now called "My Plate") is a reasonable representation of how to balance foods by quantity.

If I were to rank quantity in order of type I would suggest:

1) Non-starchy vegetable (green, leafy)
2) Protein
3) Starch or starchy vegetable
4) Fruit/Dessert

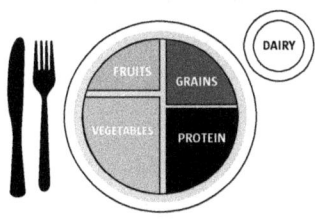

Action #7: (if applicable) Alcohol check

Throughout the entire *resetting normal* process, I did *not* give up my daily glass or two of wine with dinner. However, there is one characteristic of alcoholic beverages that can sabotage you if you're not careful: alcohol tends to release inhibitions and stimulate the appetite. Be aware of this, and if you think it's causing you to eat more than normal, drink a little less at your smaller meals.

The bottom line is that a little alcohol won't hurt your progress, but if you're pounding down a six-pack of beer or four to five cocktails every night, that will definitely sabotage your efforts. If that's your case, consider a RESET for reducing the number of alcoholic beverages. You don't have to give them up altogether, but you can probably easily get used to a few less by having water or seltzer on the table to alternate with the alcohol.

Measuring Success

Since you're not weighing in, you won't measure weight loss. But you can observe how you feel and how your clothes fit. You can *feel* lighter as you lose weight, so ask yourself how you feel each week. And if your pants are getting loose, you're losing weight. There's no time schedule to stick to; simply compare where you are with where you were one month ago.

I know everyone's in a hurry—instant gratification and all that. By comparison this may seem like a slow process, but you need to take into consideration that while it's a little slow, it's *permanent*. Once you do this—once you've reset normal—you will *never* have to do it again. Once I reset normal and got down to the appropriate size for me, my weight and size have stayed rock solid. And I can't emphasize enough how much freedom that has given me.

A caution: don't try to take it too far. Be realistic and don't aim for the Hollywood look; aim for the feeling of good health. Sometimes a relative or friend can be a good warning system. Once, in my dieting quest to get to a weight where I thought I should be, a colleague told me I'd lost so much, I looked terrible. That was certainly a wake-up call. If you've established communication with your body, you'll know when you've arrived: you'll have more energy, you won't get sick very often and your weight will be stable.

You're done!

This was the last step—the final step in *resetting normal*. Winning the four battles and conquering the final frontier does not mean you will never, ever overeat. But that's ok. As long as you listen to your internal appestat most of the time, your weight will remain stable. It's the overall average that counts, not the peaks and valleys.

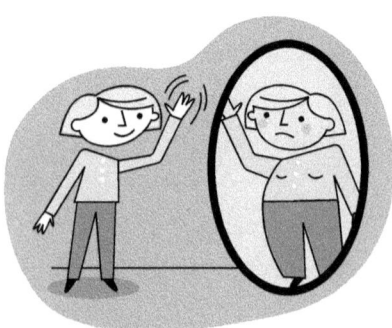

I know this must seem like an anti-climax because we are all used to the idea that losing weight is so difficult and such a big deal. But revel in the fact that you can accomplish your weight goal without engaging in a Major Project and turning your life upside down. It's easy *and* it's sustainable.

CHAPTER 12
TIPS FOR KEEPING YOUR NEW NORMAL FOREVER

Once you've gone through the entire process of *resetting normal* you shouldn't have to worry about maintenance. Remember: normal is easy to maintain—once it's established, you just do it. However, with all the pressure from outside influences, you need to be vigilant about protecting that new normal. For that purpose, I offer the following tips:

- Don't even *think* about going back to a dieting lifestyle.
- Don't be tempted to ramp up your activity routine to where you burn out—slow and steady wins the race .
- Keep up your defenses against experts. The experts may be well-intentioned, but they don't know what's going on inside your body at any given time. It doesn't mean that they are always wrong, but thoroughly evaluate every piece of advice you hear.
- Keep up your defenses against food industry marketing. Remember that their mission is to increase profit, not to make you healthy.
- Always keep a look out for new whole foods you might like, and new ways to prepare them.
- Remember the 80/20 rule: If 80 percent of what you eat is real, whole food, the other 20 percent is not going to kill you. If you want a cookie once in a while, eat it and don't beat yourself up over it—enjoy it.
- Listen to your Goldilocks moments—let them guide how much you should eat.

NOTES

PART 4: SPECIAL CASES
CHAPTER 13
HOW TO IMPROVE QUALITY ON A LIMITED BUDGET

The Context

A few times in my life I've been in a position where I didn't have to worry about how much I spent on food. But more often I've had to watch every dollar—including now, since I'm on a retirement income. So I'm very aware of the obstacles to buying quality food instead of the processed variety. In this section I would like to propose a few suggestions based on my experience.

If your income is unlimited you can buy all kinds of pricey organic, local farm-raised foods, from fresh fruits and vegetables to dairy products to grass-fed meats, and fresh, wild fish. But you don't have to go to that extreme to reset normal. You can do it with ordinary foods you find at your local supermarket; you just have to know what will give you the most bang for your buck, and you have to increase your resistance to cheap processed foods.

The prices for whole foods vary widely by region, state, community, season, and store. They also vary week to week, depending on multiple factors, including store sales. So there's no way I can recommend specific food choices based on price. I can only speak about relative cost and benefits of different food items.

IT'S HARD TO ARGUE WITH ...

The appeal of most processed foods is that they're cheap, at least on a per-calorie basis: you get a lot of calories for your money. They're also convenient and kids love them. If you're on a limited budget and you need to fill up your family, I can see how tempting fast food and frozen entrees and snacks can be. Burgers and fries, chicken nuggets, tacos, burritos, and pizza from fast-food restaurants are quick and easy and cheap. Same with their equivalent frozen counterparts in the supermarket.

But considering the adverse long-term health effects of a constant diet of these foods, if you really care about that, it's worth investing a little time and effort to replace many them with whole foods. It *is* possible to make real, whole foods inexpensively with a little attention and practice. Remember, with *Resetting Normal* you don't throw out all your current foods and habits at once, you tackle changes one at a time. That gives both you and your family time to find what you like and adjust to it.

I know it's hard to argue with convenience and price, but the end result is worth it.

THE FARMERS' MARKET IDEAL

In recent years there's been a renaissance in local farmers markets. I'm super happy about that because there's nothing better than locally raised food. But I do recognize that in our current economy it represents an ideal—an ideal that, unfortunately, not everyone can participate in. While these markets are wonderful, they are expensive. That's not because the farmers are raking in a ton of money; it simply reflects the *actual cost* of raising real food. The efficiency of our industrialized food system and government subsidies for certain products keeps prices ridiculously low compared to the rest of the world. And we've become quite used to those prices—who wouldn't? Consequently, seeing what the real price is triggers sticker shock.

For example, one time at our local farmers market I picked out three apples. When the attendant rang up the total it came to over seven dollars. I was too stunned to do anything other than pay for them. But as I walked away I couldn't help calculating that I had just paid more than two dollars for each apple. I'm sure the farmer deserved that price—the apples tasted divine—but I was careful not to do that again. Other examples: one farm-raised chicken can cost as much as thirty dollars or more, and a dozen fresh eggs easily exceeds seven dollars. I can well understand that prices like these are unsustainable for the average income and completely out of reach for a low income.

That doesn't mean you won't be able to find anything at farmers markets, though, so even if you're in a low income-bracket, give it a try. But if there's nothing there you can afford, *do not worry about it*. It may be an ideal, but people can and do live long and healthy lives on food they buy at their local supermarket. And one of the great side effects of the popularity of farmers markets is that many supermarkets are including locally produced foods in their produce section, at reasonably competitive prices.

INEXPENSIVE WHOLE FOODS

There are actually many whole foods that are relatively inexpensive.

Beans and lentils. Here's what's great about beans and lentils:

- They're high in protein, fiber, and other nutrients.
- They're filling.
- There are dozens of varieties.
- They mix well with a wide variety of spices, whole grains (pasta, cornmeal, rice, etc.), beef, pork, sausage, chicken, lamb, tofu, and vegetables.

- They come canned or dried.
- They're cheap, especially considering the food value they provide.

The canned ones are convenient, but it's cheaper if you buy dried beans and cook them yourself. A couple dollars' worth of dried beans will probably yield eight to ten cups of cooked beans, while you'd be lucky to get a quarter of that from two dollars' worth of canned beans. And if you cook a bunch at a time, you can keep them in the fridge for several meals.

Whole grain. Whole grains cost more than their refined counterparts. But there isn't *that* much difference if you don't go for the exotic varieties. Keep in mind that whole foods are more filling and you can get by with less. I've also noticed that as some of these have become more mainstream the price has come down.

Canned tomatoes. Despite information I read in the book *Tomatoland*[19] by Barry Estabrook, who describes in detail the detrimental practices used in the growth and harvesting process for canned tomatoes, I still use them frequently. If there were a reasonable alternative I'd use it, but there isn't. They're inexpensive and versatile, and I think the nutrition pluses outweigh the process minuses. You can use canned tomatoes to enhance beans, other vegetables, and meats, and for sauces.

Vegetables. The best way to buy fresh vegetables is when they're in season and when your local supermarket has them on sale. Lettuce, carrots, broccoli, cabbage, onions, potatoes, yams, and hot peppers seem to be the cheapest. But there's nothing wrong with frozen vegetables. They are picked, cleaned, and flash-frozen so quickly after harvest that they probably retain most of their nutrition.

Fruits. Same as vegetables, they're best bought in season. Out of season they're exceptionally high priced and don't taste very good. Fruits that seem to be the least expensive include bananas, apples, and oranges, although in season, watermelon is usually a great buy. There's also nothing wrong with frozen fruits in terms of nutrition, as long as they aren't frozen with sugar. However, defrosted frozen fruit tend to turn to mush, so it's better to add it to something else. Frozen fruit works great in hot and cold cereals and mixed with plain yogurt.

Proteins. One of the least expensive sources of protein is eggs. They were given a bad rap back in the 1980s and 90s, but there's been plenty of evidence since then that there's nothing wrong with eating them. For other proteins, shop the sales. Chicken and the cheaper cuts of beef, pork, and lamb tend to be the most common. Even tofu goes on sale from time to time.

Fats. Olive oil may seem expensive, but you don't need much of it so it can last a long time. It's cheaper in larger quantities and can be refrigerated. But be sure to buy it in a dark bottle or can, as light causes oils to deteriorate. Avoid frying foods not only because it's not the best food preparation, but because it requires a lot of oil and even the cheapest variety is costly. And it's not a good idea to reuse it, as it deteriorates with each use. That's one of the reasons that I rarely deep-fry anything. Peanut oil is best for high temperatures but more expensive than vegetable oil, although sometimes it's reasonably priced in stores that carry a wide range of Asian foods. I see butter on sale all the time. It's another fat to use sparingly, but at least it's a whole food.

Spices. Spices can be expensive, but they enable you to create a wide variety of different tasting dishes and keep you and your family from same-food-boredom. One way to get around the expense is to buy just one new spice per month. And you don't need the exotic ones; the basics will give you a lot to work with.

Basics: granulated or powered onion, granulated or powered garlic, oregano, basil, thyme, rosemary, chili powder, cayenne, red pepper flakes, and cumin.

Snack foods. The cheapest snack food is popcorn (unadulterated by additives), especially if you buy a bag of it and cook it yourself instead of getting microwave packages. However, if you're worried about the safety of your kids tackling this by themselves, the microwave bags work.

WHOLE FOODS THAT ARE HARD TO FIND AT A LOW PRICE

Finding good quality food like those below at a low price, while difficult and sometimes seasonally driven, is not impossible. It just may take more searching to find them.
- Whole-grain bread
- Fresh fish
- Nuts
- Fresh tomatoes
- Fresh berries

HELPFUL EQUIPMENT

You are well set if you have a couple different sizes of skillets, a Dutch oven or soup pot, some casserole pans, and a mixer. Be wary of cheap non-stick pans—they're easily scratched and as the coating comes off you'll be eating bits of it along with the food. Even if you can afford only one, get one that is hard-anodized.

One of the most useful tools, however, is the lowly slow cooker. With a slow cooker you can easily make those meal-stretching bean dishes and have them ready when you get home from work. If you can't afford a new one, you might find a used one at a place like Goodwill.

The Challenges

LIMIT PRODUCTS WITH LITTLE NUTRITIONAL VALUE

One way to free up more money for the good stuff is to limit products you really don't need. I've already talked at length about processed foods to replace, and if you're resetting normal, you're on a path to do that anyway. But as a reminder, if you don't buy soda, bottled water, gallons of fruit juice, lunch meats, too many snack foods, and too much sweet stuff, you'll free up money to buy foods that really make a difference.

I'm not suggesting that you never buy those items, just that you limit them. I know that's especially hard if you have kids. They think soda is one of the main food groups, and if they have friends over they're not going to want to offer them carrot sticks for a snack. Popcorn is a great snack if you don't buy the kind with the artificial butter-flavored goop on it; there are quality alternatives and they're cheaper anyway. Don't think of this as deprivation. Even if you have the money, you should limit these items.

Action #1: Estimate your savings

Take one week's food budget and estimate how much you spent on non-nutritious food. Then make a list of quality foods you could have bought instead. You might be surprised.

STRETCH YOUR DOLLARS

If you live on a low-income budget, I'm sure you are no stranger to what are commonly called meal stretchers: beans, lentils, corn, pasta, rice or other whole grains, cheese, and eggs.

Action #2: Try some whole-food meal stretchers

Instead of using boxed meal-fillers, you can quickly make satisfying whole-food-dishes by using canned beans, tomatoes, and frozen vegetables. Sauté onions and garlic in olive oil, add the protein of your choice, then dump everything else in, let it simmer for fifteen to twenty minutes, and call it done. Top it with cheese. Your own, personal meat helper. A big pot of soup with these ingredients is good too. Especially served with whole-grain bread or homemade cornbread and butter. You don't have to be a gourmet chef and spend a lot of money to prepare delicious foods yourself. For suggestions *see Appendix A: Whole-food alternatives.*

MANAGING WITH AN EXTREMELY LOW INCOME

I understand from talking to social services professionals that a lack of even the most basic equipment is a real problem for those who struggle with a super-low income. Some people don't have access to a proper stove or even have a place to put one. Some may not have a refrigerator large enough to store food for more than a couple of days and have limited freezer space. If you're in this category, you need more information than I can provide here. But don't give up hope—there's help out there. Just try the next Action.

Action #3: Investigate helpful resources

Surprisingly enough, the USDA, on its website, has set up some useful recipe resources for low-income budgets. Go to *usda.gov* website, enter "recipe finder" in the search field and you'll find links to low-cost recipes.

The recipes I checked looked both tasty and simple. My only reservation is that the site's cost breakdown for recipes must represent some kind of national average. Where I live, it would cost me considerably more to make them than what the USDA has specified. I'm sure it varies rather widely across the country. Still, it's a good place to go for ideas.

I realize those of you dealing with a tight food budget probably already know and do what I've outlined here, so my suggestions may seem like I'm preaching to the choir. But what I wanted to emphasize by including this small section is that I truly believe there is a way to reset normal even on a limited budget. It might not be as easy as for someone who has unlimited resources. But it is possible.

NOTES

CHAPTER 14
RESETTING NORMAL FOR KIDS

The Context

There is a flood of publicity today about the rate of obesity in children. Some estimate it at around 33 percent, although I'm not sure I believe that figure; I've grown dubious about studies and statistics from my research for this book. In any case, though, there are many overweight children and quite a public debate what to do about it.

I realize that I cannot do justice to this topic in a single chapter. It's not a simple problem and deserves a book of its own. But I do have some observations and recommendations from my own experience: I was overweight most of my childhood, and all three of my offspring grew up with weight problems. They're still fighting the side-effects as adults. While this

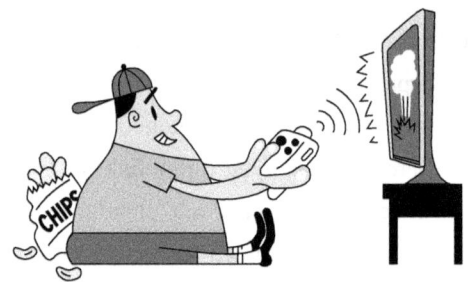

chapter is a brief overview, if your children have a weight problem, perhaps some of my ideas will help.

CONSIDER THE CHILD'S POINT OF VIEW

If you are an adult with a weight problem you know how difficult it is to fix. Earlier in this book I summarized how we got here, what is responsible, and what challenges we face. Our Western lifestyle is a direct path to obesity. Normal is not what it should be for supporting health and we face a constant barrage of noise from experts and from marketing that obscures a life-long solution.

Now consider what it's like to be a child with that problem. All those challenges are exaggerated when you're a kid because you don't have the perspective of the bigger picture; you only see what's put in front of you and you act accordingly.

CONSIDER THE FOLLOWING FROM THE CHILD'S POINT OF VIEW:
- I don't feel good about myself because my peers make fun of me and the adult authorities at school tell me I'm too fat.
- I get my perceptions of what and how much to eat from the adults around me, and they eat a lot.
- I'm told to eat my vegetables, but on the TV I see other kids eating

- candy, sweet cereals, pizza, and other fast foods.
- In my school there are vending machines with soda and junk-food snacks.
- My school lunch used to include fast-food items, and now it's nothing but stuff I don't like and there's not enough of it to fill me up.
- I have to sit in class for hours at a time and breaks for recess keep getting shorter.
- If I don't eat what the other kids are eating they make fun of me.
- I don't have a lot of self-control yet—if I can choose between carrots and a cookie I'm going to take the cookie.
- After school I have homework which keeps me sitting more.
- I like to play video games and participate in social media—if I don't I won't have any friends.
- When I'm participating in a sport, after-game treats are at a fast-food restaurant.

The environment society has created for our kids is a disaster. The trendy word for it is *obesogenic* but in a nutshell that just means we overload children with low-quality, high-calorie food and take away opportunities for an active lifestyle. Scientists engage in study upon study to try to figure out why so many kids are becoming overweight or obese. What's responsible? How can we fix it? Maybe we should classify obesity as a disease. It's a disease all right—*not a disease of the individual, though, but a disease of our society.*

WELL, DUH ...

Personally, I don't see any mystery about it. What do we expect when ...
- From the age of six months kids are exposed to advertising for junk foods like sweetened cereals, candy and fast foods.
- We use TV, movies, video games, and other sedentary-promoting devices as babysitters.
- We live sedentary lives ourselves, setting the example.
- We allow junk vending machines into schools.
- We reduce recess and physical education time.
- We live in neighborhoods where people stay mostly indoors.
- We give conflicting messages about what and how much to eat.
- We reward kids with sweet treats.
- We buy soda by the case.

- We accept supersized everything as normal.
- We're so time-strapped we rely frequently on pre-processed meals and fast-food restaurants.
- We cave in and buy the junk foods marketed to children so they don't feel left out.
- Restaurants serve the worst foods for kids.
- We design school policies that foster obesity (*rwjf.org* and search for "2009 improving child nutrition policy").

If I wanted to encapsulate this in a formula it would be:

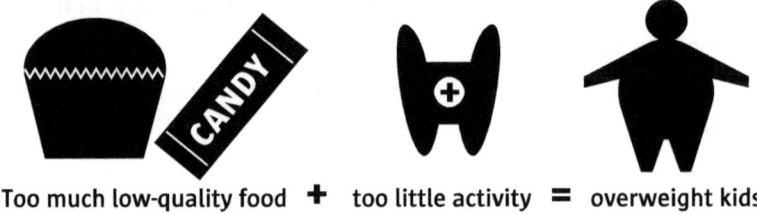

Too much low-quality food **+** too little activity **=** overweight kids

The Challenges

If you reset your normal, your children will benefit too. Start early enough, quietly and without fanfare so it isn't a shocking change they'll want to rebel against, and they'll adopt it as their normal as well—eventually. Peer pressure may make them stray, but they'll come back to it later in life. More specifically, here are a few things I would do if I had a second chance. I'll be the first to admit that none of these things is easy, but they are doable at least to some degree.

THINK LONG-TERM

We may feel that setting a good example is futile, but it isn't; it's just that sometimes it's a long-term investment. Our children might grumble and complain and even disobey, but eventually, when they're grown up, they'll see that we were right.

Action #1: Set an example

If your child is overweight, take a hard look at your family's general eating and activity habits. Don't expect your child to avoid junk food if you eat it. Expect your child to become a soda addict—regular or diet—if you buy it by the case and drink a lot of it yourself. Don't expect your child to be active if you spend most of your time sitting on the couch watching TV or surfing the internet. Be active *as a family.*

You need to be the leader.

ACT LIKE WHOLE FOODS ARE THE NORM

Feed them whole foods as often as you can. Whole foods will fill them up and last them longer. Don't let your kids make all the food decisions. They don't know what they're doing yet and they're highly likely to choose industrialized foods because they're soft, smooth, sweet, and salty, don't require much chewing, and everybody else is eating them.

A good whole-grain bread is chewy, but try to get them to eat it, even if you need to trim the crust off or cut it into fun shapes with a cookie cutter. Do everything you can to lead them away from refined carbohydrates and processed foods.

Action #2: Help them learn by doing

Help them learn to prepare whole foods themselves, not just open a package and stick it into the microwave. Kids love to do things themselves, so try to find a little time to teach them.

Desserts like cookies, cakes, and pies can be whole foods, but put more emphasis on entrée items and fruit. Avoid the mistake that I made: I thought I was doing the right thing by making my goodies from scratch but I was keeping too many of them around. In retrospect, I'd still do that once in a while, but I'd mostly provide fruit for snacks.

School lunches have been terrible in the past but are in the process of change. Support school lunch changes by serving similar whole foods at home so your kids get used to them.

SHAPE THEIR PERCEPTIONS

Action #3: Shape their perceptions in a healthy way

- Try not to create an environment of quantity. Serve reasonable portions and don't pressure them to eat more than they want.
- Don't use food as a reward or punishment. Avoid the strategies of, "If you're good you can have a cookie." or "If you don't behave yourself you can't have dessert tonight." Instead, give them a trip to the park or a new coloring book—something non-food-related.

DE-SUGARIZE THEM

Action #4: Don't get them hooked on sugar

You can do this by putting a fence around sweet foods. Make it ok to have a special sweet treat or dessert—a piece of candy or a cookie is fine once in a while—but not to have sugar in everything. That means hold your ground against sweetened cereals, frozen pastries, and anything else like that. They might make a fuss, but they'll live. No one needs to start their day with a dose of sugar, and it just gets them used to having that taste all the time. Instead, get them used to whole fruit (not just juice)—it's plenty sweet by itself.

When you feed children sweetened cereals and pastries (Toaster Strudel, Pop Tarts, etc.) for breakfast, they come to associate breakfast with sweet. It would be better to have plain cereal with fruit or whole-wheat toast with a little jam. Or set aside time to get them a small cinnamon roll or ice cream on the weekend as a treat. This builds a fence around when it's appropriate to have something sweet: not all the time, but sometimes. They'll learn that it tastes better anyway when they haven't had it for a while. If you get your kids used to the good stuff, they're more likely to develop better taste discrimination—if not right away, then later in life.

Keeping them from getting hooked on sugar also means avoiding other common foods loaded with sugar, like certain brands of peanut butter and single-serving yogurts. A yogurt product isn't necessarily healthy just because it's got yogurt in it. Read the labels; most processed foods aimed at kids have an unhealthy dose of sugar or artificial sweetener.

And especially, don't let kids drink soda like it's water. Soda is super sweet and does nothing except perpetuate a craving for sugar. Push water instead.

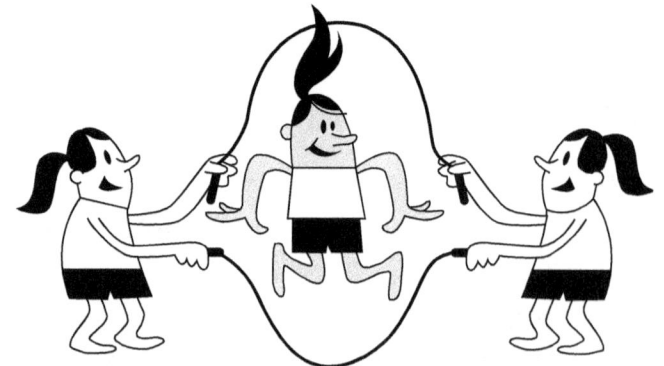

Finally, get them to expect fruit for dessert except on special occasions.

DIET-PROOF YOUR KIDS

Action #5: Don't diet

Don't diet yourself, and don't encourage them to either. It's nothing but a path to yo-yobesity, and it's so much better to set an example by eating well normally all the time.

COMMERCIAL-PROOF YOUR KIDS

There's no question that advertisers target kids directly and indirectly through their parents. Commercial-proof yourself first and then help your kids with it.

Action #6: Teach critical thinking

Teach them to be critical thinkers. I don't object to marketing—I like to know what products are out there, especially changed and new ones—but everyone should understand that the object of marketing is to convince you to buy something, not necessarily to tell the truth. Talk to your kids about the commercials, and ask them what they think is true and what's false. Ask them what they believe. Teach them how facts can be twisted and manipulated to make people believe something that's not true. Show them how to find out the truth so they can apply their own judgment in the future.

BE AN ACTIVE FAMILY

Set an example for activity as well. Don't let your kids sit for hours in front of the TV or computer. I lived in a neighborhood where my kids could go outside by themselves and run around, but there aren't many places like that anymore. If I were raising kids today I'd have to be more proactive about getting them moving.

Action #7: Find activities you can do together

Take walks together, go biking, go to the park, or basically engage in any activity that gets them up and going.

Action #8: Encourage walking and fun physical activities

Try not to drive them everywhere.
A lot of kids today hate walking, and I think it's because they're not used to having to do it. Walking is one of the best activities you can do, and if you can get them used to it, it will serve them well for their entire lives.

Encourage kids' natural inclination to be physically active: find times and safe spaces for them to jump around, climb, kick a ball, swing their arms, and try to defy gravity. The lighter they are, the easier this is for them, but help them to be as active as they can.

DO WHAT YOU CAN

Action #9: Accept your limitations

Accept that you can't control everything. It's popular today to blame the parents for an overweight child. While some might be guilty as charged, most are not. Most parents want to help, but it's very hard to figure out what to do. This entire book has been about how the whole diet approach can backfire, and that's just as true for children as adults. As a parent, I did my best to help my children lose weight. It never worked, but that was not for a lack of trying, which pre-dated my discovery of *resetting normal*.

Unless you lock your kids in the house until they're eighteen, there are going to be a lot of influences in their lives that you can't control. You might monitor what movies they see at home, but when they go to their friends' houses, the permissions could be entirely different. Likewise, you can't monitor everything they eat. All you can do is control what you can and set a good example. Just keep the 80/20 rule in mind: a little of the processed stuff won't hurt them and will keep them from becoming an outcast with their peers.

Action #10: Do the best you can

The causes of childhood obesity are the same as the causes of adulthood obesity, and that means that the solution must be similar: they must reset their normal. But they can't do this by themselves. To help them, make sure that you, as a parent, reset normal for yourself. As you go through this process, you can also nudge your family into resetting their normal because if you stop espousing the diet mindset, start serving whole foods, ramp up your activity level, and change your perceptions about quantity, your family will change as well. You won't get them to lose weight by forcibly limiting calories, fat, carbs or anything else like that; that will only drive them into the yo-yobesity pattern. It will only get done by helping them change their normal.

There have been examples in the news of some families who helped their kids lose weight, not by singling out the child with the weight problem, but by working as a whole family to change their lifestyle together. I emphatically believe that is the only long-term solution.

NOTES

PART 5: WRAPPING IT UP

I covered a lot more territory in this book than I originally intended. When I started out, I was just going to reverse-engineer how I was finally able to lose weight and maintain it, and then reconstruct it in a way that others could follow if they wanted to give it a try. I had my list of gripes about having been misled by so-called experts over many years, as I discovered how many nutritional guidelines cemented as truths in the public's minds were based on flimsy and sometimes flawed evidence. But I've tried—after much editing—to focus on what you can do about it despite all the collective brainwashing.

To achieve what I did in *Resetting Normal* I had to ignore those guidelines and come up with my own. Had it not worked so astonishingly well, I would not be recommending that you do the same. I am sure many experts will object to the lack of specific weight-loss goals in this plan. They will claim that without those, there can be no accountability. I will argue that the goals I propose are better because they are achievable. You cannot guarantee that you will lose a certain number of pounds within a given time. But if you set a goal to eat one meal of whole foods a week, you *can* make that happen. If you set a goal to walk ten minutes a day three times a week, you can make that happen.

Winning The War completely changed my life. Pre-war, my life revolved around an obsession with food and dieting. Up the scale, down the scale, up, down, over-and-over—classic yo-yobesity. Post-war, I enjoy food without the obsession, and I can focus on higher, more meaningful life goals.

Life without yo-yobesity is fantastic! No mo' yo-yo!

NOTES

APPENDIX A: WHOLE-FOOD ALTERNATIVES

Resetting Normal is not a recipe book, but in case you need help figuring out how to replace low-quality, processed foods with high-quality whole foods, this section includes a few recipes and techniques to get you started. I will gradually be adding more recipes on the companion website ***resettingnormal.com***.

RECIPE BOOKS

There are thousands of recipes available in books, magazines, and online. While it's great to have that many choices, it can be overwhelming. To mitigate this problem, when you're searching, quickly scan the recipes and eliminate any that include too many processed ingredients. I don't always have time to hunt through all the options so I have a few recipe books I rely on for both everyday and entertaining meals. Here are five of my favorites.

> Martha Stewart Living Omnimedia, Inc. *Fresh Flavor Fast: 250 easy, delicious recipes for any time of day*. New York: Clarkson Potter/Publishers, 2010.
>
> Simmons, Marie. *Fresh & Fast: Inspired Cooking for Every Season and Every Day*. Shelburne, VT: Chapters Publishing Ltd., 1996.
>
> Weil, Andrew, M.D and Rosie Daley. *The Healthy Kitchen: Recipes for a Better Body, Life, and Spirit*. New York: Alfred A. Knopf, 2002.
>
> Madison, Deborah. *Vegetable Soups from Deborah Madison's Kitchen*. New York: Broadway Books, 2006.
>
> Robertson, Robin. *Fresh from the Vegetarian Slow Cooker*. Boston: The Harvard Common Press, 2004.

SEASONINGS

Seasoning is the secret to creating great-tasting whole foods. Most of the single-ingredient spices available in the supermarket are fine, but a lot of the combination seasonings have undesirable additives or unidentified ingredients. There are basic spices you can keep on hand to create a wide variety of your own combinations. All you need to do is stock your pantry with them and experiment.

But you don't have to create all your spice combinations from scratch. There are a few spice companies that have both the basic spices and their own proprietary mixes—all without additives and preservatives. My go-to spice company is Penzeys Spices and they can be found at *penzeys.com*. They have a few brick-and-mortar stores around the country, but I order mine online, and depending on the order quantity or a special promotion, shipping can be free.

In some of the recipes that follow, I specify the Penzeys spice mix that I use, but also include a list of the individual ingredients in that mix. Penzeys does not divulge the proportion of the ingredients (for proprietary reasons) but if you don't want to order their spices, you can try to approximate with a similar combination.

You can find other sources of unadulterated spices, such as Morton & Bassett (*mortonbassett.com*) and Simply Organic (*simplyorganic.com*) in most supermarkets. Trader Joe's has a reasonable selection, and Tom Douglas's Rub with Love collection is excellent. However, they don't have anywhere near the variety of mixes that Penzeys does, even online. In selecting spices—as always, check the label—the thing to watch for is a product ingredient list that includes unspecified items. For instance, Simply Organic's Adobo Seasoning lists the main ingredients but adds, " ... along with several other supporting spices." Those "supporting spices" may be perfectly fine, but how would you know for sure?

BASIC SEASONINGS

There are dozens of different spices, but if you just start with the basic dry seasonings below, you can add one at a time as you expand your repertoire.

For savory dishes:
- Black pepper
- Granulated onion (or powdered, without salt)
- Granulated garlic (or powdered, without salt)
- Oregano
- Basil
- Thyme
- Rosemary
- Chili powder
- Red pepper flakes
- Cumin
- Mild (or sweet) curry powder
- Italian seasoning
- Cayenne pepper (if you like spicy)

For baked goods:
- Vanilla (real, not vanillin)
- Cinnamon
- Ginger

HANDY MIXES FROM SCRATCH

Two of the most useful combination seasonings are Italian and Mexican (also called Adobo) seasoning. If you can't find a satisfactory version of Italian seasoning or Adobo, here are two recipes for mixing your own.

Italian Seasoning

INGREDIENTS
- 3 Tablespoons dried basil
- 3 Tablespoons dried oregano
- 3 Tablespoons dried parsley flakes
- 1 Tablespoon granulated or powdered garlic
- 1 teaspoon dried thyme
- 1 teaspoon dried rosemary, crushed
- ¼ teaspoon black pepper

DIRECTIONS
1) Put all ingredients in a small bowl and mix well, crushing a little with something small and flat, such as the bottom of a shot glass, or with your fingers
2) Store in an airtight container for up to three months.

Mexican Adobo

INGREDIENTS
- 1 Tablespoon salt
- 1 Tablespoon paprika
- 2 teaspoons ground black pepper
- 1½ teaspoons granulated or powdered onion
- 1½ teaspoons dried oregano
- 1½ teaspoons ground cumin
- 1 teaspoon granulated or powdered garlic
- 1 teaspoon chili powder

DIRECTIONS
1) In a bowl, stir together all ingredients
2) Store in an airtight container for up to three months.

EASY WHOLE GRAINS

PASTA

Whole-wheat pasta might take just a little longer to cook than the white, refined variety, but you can use it in the same recipes.

PILAF FROM SCRATCH

While there are some boxed pilafs that don't have mysterious ingredients, a whole-grain pilaf is simple to make from scratch. If the whole grain is already cooked, it's barely a ten-minute process. These days, you can find pre-cooked whole grains in the store, on the shelf or in the freezer. If those aren't available in your area, below are some basic proportions and cooking times. You can always cook them ahead when you have time and refrigerate for quick access.

Common whole grains are brown rice, bulgur (cracked wheat), quinoa and barley. The basic cooking method is to bring the liquid (water or broth) to boil (with/without salt), add the grain, and cook over lowest heat until water is absorbed. Once the grain is cooked, you can use it plain, in soups, or as a pilaf.

- Brown rice: 2 cups liquid, 1 cup rice; cook for 50 minutes (makes 2 cups rice).
- Bulgur/cracked wheat: 2 cups liquid, 1 cup bulger; cook for 15—20 minutes and let stand for 10 minutes.
- Quinoa: 2 cups liquid, 1 cup quinoa; cook for 10—15 minutes.
- Barley: 2½ cups liquid, 1 cup barley; cook for 35—40 minutes.

Basic Pilaf

Makes 2 cups

Takes only about 10 minutes: 5 minutes to prep and 5 minutes to sauté and heat.

INGREDIENTS

- 2 cups cooked whole grain
- 2 Tablespoons olives oil
- 1 clove garlic, minced
- ¼ teaspoon dried thyme or Italian seasoning
- ¼ teaspoon red pepper flakes (optional)
- ½ cup chopped scallions
- Salt and pepper to taste

DIRECTIONS

1) Put olive oil in a medium flat sauce pan over medium heat.
2) Add garlic, thyme, scallions, and red pepper (if using)

3) Cook for 2—3 minutes, stirring a couple of times.

4) Add whole grain and stir to mix until heated through.

5) Add salt and pepper to taste.

BREAKFAST IDEAS

CEREALS

Most cold breakfast cereals contain too much sugar and artificial flavorings. You can avoid this by sticking to the basic ones (such as Shredded Wheat, Wheaties, plain Cheerios, etc.) and adding your own flavorings and fruit—it only takes a minute.

A couple of suggestions:
- ½ cup fruit: sliced banana, blueberries (frozen or fresh), other berries, or fresh fruit in season
- 2 Tablespoons chopped dried fruit
- ½ teaspoon cinnamon
- 2 Tablespoons sliced, slivered, or chopped nuts of your choice (almonds, walnuts, pecans).
- If you can't stand cereal without any sweetener, add one teaspoon sugar. That's less than most processed cereals and at least you have control of how much you add.

For hot cereals, use plain oatmeal instead of the instant—it only takes a few minutes to cook in the microwave. Or, if you want to try a wheat cereal, Krusteaz makes one called Zoom that has only one ingredient—100 percent whole wheat—and it cooks in only one minute. Flavor the hot cereals the same as for the cold ones above.

SOUTHWEST BREAKFAST MUFFINS

These muffins/squares are mostly eggs and cheese, with just enough flour to hold them together. They're great for breakfast because you can make a batch, freeze them, and then heat one or two briefly in the microwave for an instant breakfast or lunch protein.

Makes 12 regular-sized muffins or one 8 x 8 pan

INGREDIENTS
- 5 eggs
- 1 cup cottage cheese

- ½ cup whole-wheat pastry flour (or all-purpose unbleached flour)
- ½ teaspoon baking powder
- 2 Tablespoons flax oil (or corn or other vegetable oil)
- ½ teaspoon salt
- 2 Tablespoons minced green onions
- 1 4-oz can chopped green chilies (mild or hot), drained
- 2 cups grated Monterey Jack cheese

DIRECTIONS

1) Pre-heat oven to 350 degrees.

2) Spray 12-muffin pan or square baking pan with Pam.

   **Note: don't use cupcake papers because the egg muffin will stick to them.

3) In a large bowl:

   a. Beat the eggs.

   b. Add cottage cheese.

   c. Beat until almost smooth.

   d. Beat in flour, baking powder, and flax oil until thoroughly blended.

   e. Stir in onions, chilies, and cheese.

4) To bake muffins:

   a. Divide mixture into 12 muffin spaces.

   b. Bake 30 minutes. Muffins should be firm in the center when done.

   c. Let cool slightly.

   d. Using a small metal spatula, loosen muffins and remove to a cooling rack.

5) To bake in pan:

   a. Pour mixture into pan.

   b. Bake 35—40 minutes.

   c. Let cool slightly.

   d. Cut into desired serving sizes.

6) To freeze for later individual use:

   a. When cool, put in a plastic bag or container and freeze.

   b. To serve, heat in microwave.

FLAVOR-YOUR-OWN YOGURT

Instead of pre-sweetened yogurt, try this:

INGREDIENTS

- ¾ cup plain whole yogurt (or Greek yogurt, if you prefer). Whole yogurt

is much less tart than the low- or non-fat varieties so it doesn't demand extra sweeteners.
- ½ cup sliced or chopped fresh or defrosted frozen fruit (bananas, berries, peaches, apples)
- ½ teaspoon cinnamon—adds sweetness without sugar
- 2 Tablespoons sliced, slivered, or chopped nuts of your choice (almonds, walnuts, pecans)
- 2 Tablespoons plain, unsweetened (or very lightly sweetened). crunchy cereal, such as Grape Nuts

DIRECTIONS

1) In serving bowl, mix yogurt with cinnamon.
2) Add the remaining ingredients and mix.

SALAD DRESSINGS

It's hard to find a bottled salad dressing with quality ingredients. Besides additives, preservatives, and a lot of sugar, most are based on canola, soy, or other cheap oil rather than olive oil. The best ones are in the refrigerated section of the market, but they're expensive and don't keep for a long time. Instead, you can whip up a quick salad dressing as you go, in only a few minutes.

Here are three salad dressing recipes. In each case, add the minimum amount of dressing, toss thoroughly, and add only one tablespoon more at a time—tossing after each addition—until all the ingredients are lightly coated and there is no large pool of dressing in the bottom.

OIL & VINEGAR DRESSING

One of the easiest salad dressings to make is oil and vinegar. It only takes a few minutes, so I usually make it when I prepare the salad.
Dressing for about 4 cups salad greens (4 small or 2 large servings)

INGREDIENTS
- 1 Tablespoon olive oil
- 1 teaspoon prepared Dijon mustard
- 1 teaspoon Italian seasoning, with or without salt
- ¼ teaspoon salt (if Italian seasoning is unsalted)
- 1 teaspoon vinegar (Balsamic, wine, cider, white, or rice)

DIRECTIONS

1) Put Italian seasoning in small bowl with 1 Tablespoon water, let sit for 5 minutes.
2) Add olive oil, mustard, vinegar and salt (if using).
3) Whisk until well blended.

OIL & LEMON JUICE DRESSING

This is a variation of oil and vinegar. It works well as an accompaniment to a heavier richer dinner, as it's very light.

Dressing for about 4 cups salad greens (4 small or 2 large servings)

INGREDIENTS

- 2 Tablespoons olive oil
- Pinch of salt
- Pepper to taste
- 1 Tablespoon lemon juice

DIRECTIONS

1) Put olive oil in small bowl.
2) Add lemon juice and salt and whisk till blended.
3) Add pepper to taste.

RANCH-STYLE DRESSING

Makes one cup dressing

INGREDIENTS

- ½ cup Mayonnaise
- ½ cup Buttermilk
- 1 Tablespooon Penzeys Buttermilk Ranch Dressing Base
  (or *alternative seasoning mix* below)

DIRECTIONS

1) Put Buttermilk Ranch Dressing Base seasoning in small bowl with 1 Tablespoon water, let sit for 5 minutes.
2) Add mayonnaise and whisk to blend.
3) Slowly add buttermilk, whisking until well-blended.
4) Store in refrigerator (up to a week) and whisk or shake well before serving.

ALTERNATIVE SEASONING MIX

- ½ teaspoon granulated or powdered garlic
- ½ teaspoon granulated or powdered onion

- 1 teaspoon Italian seasoning or boquet garni
- ¼ teaspoon salt (if Italian seasoning is unsalted)

UN-BOXED DINNERS

Boxed dinners may seem convenient, but it really doesn't take that much longer to put one together yourself. Instead, try one of these.

GROUND MEAT DINNER

INGREDIENTS

- 1 lb. ground meat—beef, turkey, chicken, pork, or lamb
- 2 Tablespoons olive oil
- ½ cup chopped large onion (about ½ large or 1 medium)
- 2 cloves garlic (chopped or pressed)
- 1 15-oz. can beans—red, black, pinto, kidney (about 2 cups, with liquid)
- 1 14.5-oz. can chopped tomatoes or tomato puree
- 1 teaspoon Italian seasoning (or alternative given below)
- 1 teaspoon salt (if Italian seasoning is unsalted)
- 1 teaspoon granulated or powdered onion
- ½ teaspoon red pepper flakes (optional)
- 1 cup broth—beef, chicken or vegetable
- Pepper to taste
- 3 cups cooked pasta, such as whole-wheat elbow macaroni

DIRECTIONS

1) In wide skillet over medium heat, cook the ground meat, breaking it apart, until mostly cooked.
2) Drain off any excess fat from the meat.
3) Add olive oil.
4) Add onion and garlic, stir to mix and continue to cook until onion is softened
5) Add Italian seasoning, granulated or powdered onion, pepper flakes, salt and pepper, and cook for 1—2 minutes more.
6) Add tomatoes, beans with their liquid, and broth.
7) Bring to a simmer, turn on low and cook for about 15 minutes.
8) You can add cooked pasta; heat for a few minutes and serve; or serve the pasta separately and let individuals combine their own in the quantities they prefer.
9) A salad completes this entrée nicely.

VARIATIONS

Add one or more of the following along with the onions:
- 1 cup roughly chopped green and/or red sweet peppers
- 1 cup diced zucchini
- 1 cup peas
- 1 cup fresh sliced mushrooms, or one 7-oz. can

Instead of Italian seasoning, use the following for a Southwest flavor
- ½ teaspoon oregano
- ½ teaspoon cumin
- ½ teaspoon chili powder

TACOS

Use a standard taco preparation with condiments, but instead of a prepared packet of taco seasoning—which usually has MSG, among other additives—use the following per every pound of meat.
- 2 teaspoons Adobo seasoning
- 1 teaspoon granulated or powdered onion
- ¼ teaspoon dried oregano
- ½ teaspoon cumin
- ½ teaspoon chili powder
- 1 teaspoon salt (or to taste)
- ¼ teaspoon pepper

FISH DINNER

With fresh or frozen fish filets, you can have dinner on the table in 30 minutes.

INGREDIENTS
- Frozen or fresh fish filets (e.g., cod, Mahi-Mahi, halibut, salmon)— 6 – 8 oz. per serving
- Seasoning—choose from:
    - Salt and pepper to taste
    - ⅛ teaspoon Italian seasoning per serving and salt (if not included in seasoning)
    - Salt, pepper, and ⅛ teaspoon thyme per serving
- Squeeze of lemon juice

- Frozen string beans
- Packet of Seeds of Change frozen Quinoa and Brown Rice with Garlic

DIRECTIONS

1) If frozen, defrost fish per package instructions.
2) Cut fish into serving-size pieces, if necessary.
3) Place on broiler pan and sprinkle with seasoning.
4) Choose one method of cooking:
    a. Broil 10 minutes per 1-inch thickness of fish.
    b. Pre-heat oven to 450 degrees and bake for 15 minutes.
5) Squeeze lemon juice on top.
6) Cook string beans per package instructions (about 5 minutes).
7) Cook brown rice/quinoa per instructions (for Seeds of Change, 90 seconds in microwave).

MAC & CHEESE

Who doesn't love mac and cheese? Yes, making it from scratch isn't as quick as dumping a box in a pot, but either way you have to cook the macaroni, and the time it takes is pretty short when you use pre-grated cheese.

Easily serves 4 as a side dish—feel free to cut recipe in half or double it.

INGREDIENTS

- 2 cups pasta, about 4 oz.—preferably whole wheat (shape of your choice, although elbow macaroni is traditional)
- 2 Tablespoons butter
- 2 Tablespoons flour
- 1 teaspoon Penzeys Foxpoint seasoning (or *alternate seasoning* below)

- *Alternate seasoning:*
    o ¼ teaspoon granulated or powdered onion
    o ¼ teaspoon granulated or powdered garlic
    o ¼ teaspoon dry mustard
    o ¼ teaspoon salt
- 1½ cups whole milk
- 4 oz. shredded medium cheddar cheese
- 4 oz. shredded Monterey Jack cheese
- ¼ cup grated parmesan or Romano cheese

DIRECTIONS

1) Bring water to boil in large pot. Add pasta and cook until done, 8 to 10 minutes, depending on the shape of pasta. Test for doneness, as some people prefer al dente and others soft. Drain in colander.
2) Melt butter in 1-quart saucepan over medium heat.
3) Add 2 tablespoons flour and cook, stirring often with a whisk for about 2 minutes.
4) Add Foxpoint or Alternate seasoning, stirring for 1—2 minutes.
5) Add milk and cook, whisking often until slightly thickened (about 5 minutes).
6) Remove from heat and let cool for about 1 minute. (Adding cheddar cheese to the liquid when it's too hot can make the mixture curdle.)
7) Add grated cheese and parmesan or Romano and mix well.
8) Return pan to heat over low and stir with whisk just until cheese is melted.
9) Remove from heat.
10) Taste and add salt if necessary and pepper if desired.
11) If cooked pasta is stuck together, rinse briefly with hot water.
12) Put pasta in serving dish, add sauce, stir well and serve. If it is too thick, add a little milk and stir.

CHICKEN IN A FLASH

Boneless, skinless chicken breast cooks very quickly. This recipe takes about 10 minutes prep and 10—12 minutes cooking time.

INGREDIENTS

- Boneless, skinless chicken breast, cut into serving-size pieces of about 4 – 6 oz.
- Choose *one* of following seasonings (amount per pound of chicken):
    - Italian seasoning: 2 teaspoons
    - Adobo seasoning: 2 teaspoons
    - 1 teaspoon granulated or powdered garlic + 1 teaspoon granulated or powdered onion + salt and pepper
    - 2 teaspoons Penzeys Northwoods (salt, paprika, black pepper, thyme, rosemary, granulated or powdered garlic, and chipotle pepper)
    - 2 teaspoons Penzeys Rocky Mountain seasoning
- Salt and pepper (if not included in seasoning)
- 1 Tablespoon Olive oil
- 1 Tablespoon Butter

DIRECTIONS

1) Rub chicken pieces with seasoning.
2) Heat skillet over medium-high heat with 1 Tablespoon each olive oil and butter.
3) Put chicken pieces in skillet without crowding.
4) Cook for about 5 minutes.
5) Turn pieces and cook another 5 minutes or until white through the center.
6) If you have more pieces, cook a second round, adding a little more olive oil and butter if necessary.

EASY FAMILY SOUPS

EASY MINESTRONE

Makes about 2 quarts of soup

You can make this in a soup pot or slow cooker. Directions below are for a soup pot. To make in a slow cooker, simply do steps 1 and 2 of the directions, then put everything in the slow cooker and cook 6—8 hours.

NOTES:

- Measurements for vegetables are approximate—it really doesn't matter if you use a little over or under the amount given.
- I always put the pasta in the soup bowls when serving—otherwise it will soak up too much broth.

INGREDIENTS

Vegetables:

- 1 cup onion: large dice (about ½ large or one medium)
- 2 cloves garlic, finely chopped (about 1 Tablespoon)
- 1 stalk celery: diced (about ½ cup)
- 2 carrots: sliced (about 1 cup)
- 1 cup summer squash (zucchini or yellow): large dice
- 1 medium potato: peeled, large dice (about 1 cup)

Seasoning:

- 1 teaspoon salt
- ½ teaspoon black pepper
- 1 teaspoon Italian seasoning
- 2 teaspoons dried basil
- ½ teaspoon granulated or powered onion
- ¼ teaspoon red pepper flakes (optional: use more if you like spicy)

Additional Ingredients:
- 1 quart vegetable broth
- 1 cup shredded cabbage
- ¼ cup finely chopped parsley (optional)
- 1 cup frozen string beans
- 8 oz. can garbanzo beans (about 1 cup with liquid)
- 8 oz. can red kidney beans (about 1 cup with liquid)
- 1 cup canned chopped tomato
- ½ cup cooked pasta (your choice) per person
- Grated parmesan or Romano cheese

DIRECTIONS

1) On medium heat, sauté in 4 quart soup pot for 10 minutes:
    a. 2 Tablespoons olive oil
    b. Onion, garlic, celery, carrots, zucchini and potato
2) Add seasoning mix and sauté for 2 minutes.
3) Add:
    a. Vegetable broth
    b. Frozen string beans
    c. Shredded cabbage
    d. Tomatoes
    e. Garbanzo and kidney beans
    f. Parsley
4) Bring to boil and simmer on low for about 12 minutes, or until potatoes and zucchini are tender when pierced with a fork.
5) While soup is simmering, cook pasta in boiling water until desired doneness.

TO SERVE
- Put ½ cup pasta in soup bowl.
- Ladle soup over top.
- Sprinkle with parmesan or Romano cheese.

TIME-SAVING TIPS
- Refrigerated, peeled garlic
- Pre-cut onion and celery
- Frozen sliced carrots
- Bagged shredded cabbage

- Instead of cutting vegetables separately, use a package of frozen Italian vegetables (then you'll only have to cut the potato).

BEAN & BACON SOUP

Bean and bacon is a hearty soup that's especially good in cold weather and makes a complete meal with the addition of a salad. The following recipe is a good approximation of the canned variety. I like to make it in a slow cooker but you can also cook it in a large soup pot.

This recipe makes a lot of soup—around 3 quarts. If you don't need that much, cut the ingredients in half. But this soup freezes well, so if you want to have some handy for another dinner, make the larger quantity.

INGREDIENTS
- 6 pieces thick-sliced bacon or bacon end pieces, chopped
- 1 cup chopped onion (about ½ large or 1 medium)
- 1 stalk celery, chopped
- 2 carrots, chopped
- 2 cloves garlic, finely chopped
- 8 cups home-cooked or canned small white beans (navy, pea, or great northern) with 1 cup liquid
- 4 oz. tomato paste
- ½ teaspoon salt
- ½ teaspoon dried thyme
- 2 bay leaves
- ½ teaspoon Tabasco sauce (optional)
- About 2 cups broth (or 2 cans)—chicken, beef, or veggie

DIRECTIONS
1) Mash 2 cups of the beans in a blender, food processor, a bowl and fork, or a potato masher, and set aside
2) In a large, deep skillet over medium heat, cook chopped bacon till slightly browned but not completely dry—if this generates a lot of fat, remove all but about 1 Tablespoon.
3) Add onion, celery, garlic, and carrots and sauté until onion is translucent (about 10 minutes).
4) Stir in tomato paste and gradually add enough broth to thin it for easy mixing.
5) Put bacon and sautéed vegetables in slow cooker or large soup pot.

6) Add whole beans, mashed beans, salt, thyme, broth, and bay leaves.
7) For slow cooker, cover and cook on low 6—8 hours (precise time is not critical); for soup pot, bring to boil then simmer on low, covered, about 30 minutes.
8) When done, remove bay leaves.
9) Have more Tabasco sauce available for those who like heat.

UN-BOXED DESSERTS

Plain fruit is the best and easiest dessert, but if you want to break up the monotony, try one of these recipes. They don't take much time but each is a little different.

INTERESTING WAYS TO SERVE FRUIT
Rehydrated Apricots

Canned apricots are expensive and while fresh ones are ok in season, sometimes they're not picked when ripe and don't have much flavor. Dried apricots do have a more intense flavor and are available year-round. Once they're rehydrated, you can add a couple to hot cereal as a fruit sweetener, eat 3 or 4 for a snack, or make a quick dessert by adding ¼ cup ice cream.

INGREDIENTS
- 1 cup dried apricots

INSTRUCTIONS
1) Put apricots in a medium saucepan and add water to about 1 inch above apricots.
2) Cover and bring to a boil.
3) Remove from heat and let cool.
4) Serve warm or cold.
5) Store in refrigerator in their liquid; will keep for a couple of weeks.

Blueberry Freeze

Makes one serving at a time

INGREDIENTS
- ½ cup frozen blueberries
- ½ cup whole milk
- Dash of vanilla
- 1 teaspoon sugar (optional)

DIRECTIONS
1) Put all ingredients in a blender and blend on high until smooth.
2) Serve in a dish like ice cream.

Flavored Fruit
INGREDIENTS
- Fresh fruit such as berries, peaches or nectarines— ½ cup per serving
- Potential flavorings
    - o 1 Tablespoon Grand Marnier or other orange liqueur
    - o 1 Tablespoon Chambord (raspberry liqueur)
    - o 1 Tablespoon vanilla syrup (the type used to flavor coffee drinks)
    - o 1 Tablespoon Amaretto (almond liqueur)
    - o 1 teaspoon almond syrup (the type used to flavor coffee drinks)
- 2 Tablespoons whipped cream or vanilla ice cream (optional)

DIRECTIONS
1) Slice fruit into bowl
2) Add flavoring of choice and stir
3) Serve as is or with whipped cream or ice cream

BAKED GOODS

Generally speaking, we shouldn't eat many sweet baked goods, but there are times when it's called for. Here are a couple of one-bowl cake recipes that are fast and just as easy to make as boxed mixes.

Cocoa Cake

This cake has many great features. It mixes up in one bowl, doesn't require eggs or butter, and it's quick: ideal if you have company coming and don't have much time to prepare, or if your kid forgot to tell you they need a cake until eight in the evening. It works for either a cake or cupcakes, and it's also good with or without a little icing. Its history goes back to World War II, when eggs and butter were scarce and someone came up with a way to make a great cake without those crucial ingredients.

For cake: grease and flour an 8- or 9-inch square baking pan.

For cupcakes: this recipe makes about 1 dozen—put cupcake papers into cupcake pan.

Pre-heat oven to 350 degrees.

INGREDIENTS
- 1½ cups unsifted all-purpose flour
- 1 cup granulated sugar
- ¼ cup cocoa (unsweetened—not cocoa mix)
- 1 teaspoon baking soda
- ½ teaspoon salt
- 1 cup water
- ¼ cup plus 2 Tablespoons vegetable oil
- 1 Tablespoon vinegar (white or cider)
- 1 teaspoon vanilla

DIRECTIONS

1) In a large mixing bowl, combine flour, sugar, cocoa, baking soda, and salt.
2) Add water, vegetable oil, vinegar and vanilla.
3) Beat until smooth and thoroughly blended (by mixer or hand).
4) For cake: bake at 350 for 35—40 minutes or until cake tester (e.g. toothpick) comes out clean.
5) For cupcakes: bake at 350 for about 20 minutes.

OPTIONAL CHOCOLATE ICING

1) Right after removing cake from oven, sprinkle ¾ cup chocolate chips on top.
2) Let sit about 10 minutes to melt.
3) Spread over cake with a metal spatula.

Vanilla Cake

Here's a one-bowl all-purpose vanilla cake from scratch.

For cake: grease and flour an 8-inch square baking pan.

For cupcakes: this recipe makes about 1 dozen—put cupcake papers into cupcake pan.

Pre-heat oven to 350 degrees.

INGREDIENTS
- 1½ cups unsifted all-purpose flour
- ¾ cup sugar + ½ teaspoon salt
- 1 Tablespoon baking powder
- 1 egg
- ¾ cup whole milk

- 1 teaspoon vanilla
- 6 Tablespoons vegetable oil

DIRECTIONS

1) Put flour, sugar + salt, and baking powder in large mixing bowl and stir to combine.
2) Add egg, vanilla, and milk and beat one minute (by hand or mixer).
3) Add oil and beat one more minute.
4) For cake: bake at 350 for 30 minutes or until cake tester (e.g. toothpick) comes out clean.
5) For cupcakes: bake at 350 for about 20 minutes.

OPTIONAL CHOCOLATE ICING

1) Right after removing cake from oven, sprinkle ¾ cup chocolate chips on top.
2) Let sit about 10 minutes to melt.
3) Spread over cake with a metal spatula.

Cake Variations

You can use the basic vanilla cake recipe to make different flavors, with a few simple substitutions:

Spice Cake:
- Replace plain sugar with ¾ cup packed dark-brown sugar.
- Leave out vanilla and replace with 1 teaspoon cinnamon, ½ teaspoon ginger, and ¼ teaspoon cloves (or use 1½ teaspoons apple pie or pumpkin pie spice).

Lemon Cake:
- Replace vanilla with lemon extract.
- Add 1 Tablespoon lemon zest with egg and milk.

Orange Cake:
- Replace vanilla with orange extract.
- Add 1 Tablespoon orange zest with egg and milk.

APPENDIX B: ACTION TOOLS

SAMPLE AEROBICS TRACKING CHART

For the Battle of Activity, Action #14 (optional)

If you want to keep track of your progress, a simple activity log (such as the sample below) will suffice. You only need to create as many columns as the number of different activities you choose, but you might want to add a couple of blank columns so that if you have opportunities to do something fun and different, you can add it easily.

Date	Walk	Cycle	Stepper
Mon, 5/10/17	10 minutes		
Wed, 5/12/17	10 minutes		
Fri, 5/14/17			15 minutes
Sat, 5/15/17		30 minutes	

The advantage to a tracking chart is that you can easily see your progress timewise. If you start out at ten minutes and progress to a half hour after a couple of months, that's great. If you stall out, you can see that too, and it will remind you to correct course.

NOTES

SOME COMMON STRENGTH ACTIVITIES:

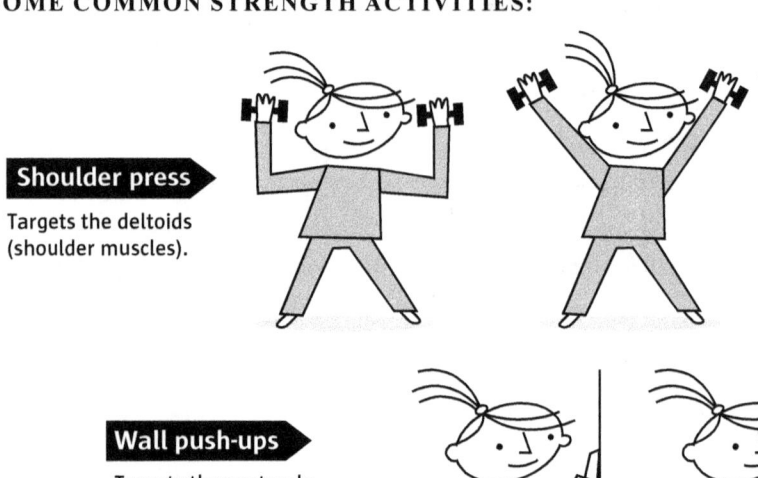

Shoulder press
Targets the deltoids (shoulder muscles).

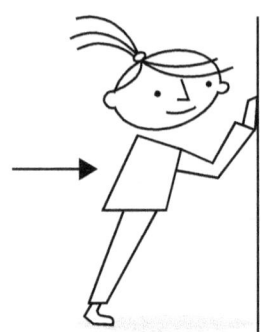
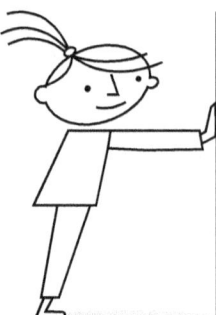

Wall push-ups
Targets the pectorals (chest muscles), triceps (rear arm muscles) and deltoids (shoulder muscles)

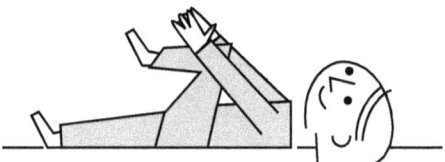

Leg raise and knee-to-chest
Targets the abductors (outer thigh muscles) and hip flexor muscles.

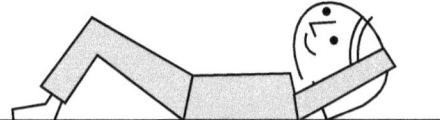

Abdominal curl-up
Targets the upper and middle abdominal muscles.

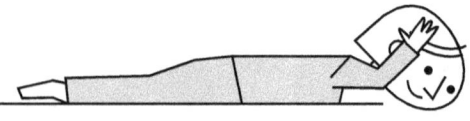

Lower back extension
Targets the back muscles and stretches the abdominals.

SOME COMMON STRENGTH ACTIVITIES:

Tricep kickback
Targets the triceps (muscles in the back of the upper arm).

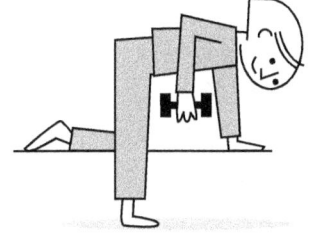
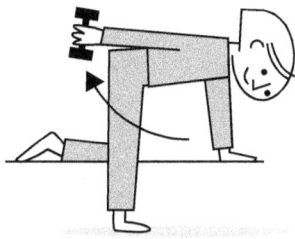

Single-arm row
Targets the latissimus dorsi (large back muscles) but also involves shoulders, arms, and abdominals.

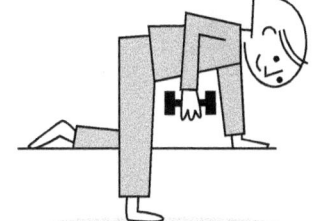
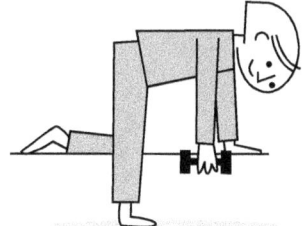

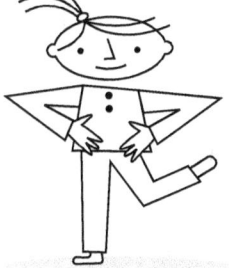

Balancing
Targets core strength, especially the quadriceps (muscles in front of the thighs).

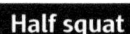

Half squat
Targets the quadriceps (front thigh muscles) and the gluteus (buttocks).

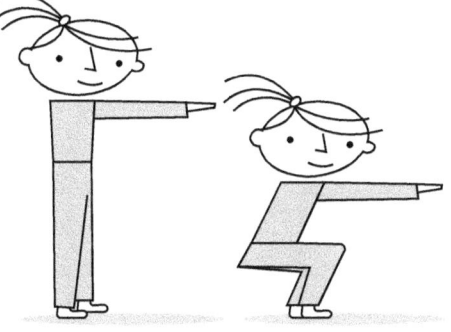

Reverse lunge
Targets the back muscles and stretches the abdominals.

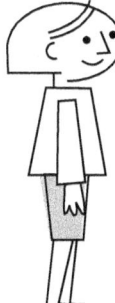
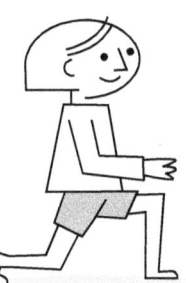

SOME COMMON STRENGTH ACTIVITIES:

Bicep curl

Targets the biceps (muscles that bend the arm).

Side bend

Targets the outer area of the abdominals (along the side).

✎ NOTES

SAMPLE STRENGTH TRAINING TRACKING CHART

For the Battle of Activity, Action #24

Consider using a chart to help you track your progress. The sample below assumes a strength workout twice a week, starting at a beginning level and increasing very gradually. (You would start each day with blank entries and fill in your actual numbers as you go.)

	Mon, 7/3/17		Thurs, 7/6/17		Mon, 7/10/17		Thurs, 7/1317		Mon, 7/17/17		Thurs, 7/20/17	
warmup	X		X		X		X		X		X	
	weight	reps	weight	reps	weight	reps	weight	reps	weight	reps	weight	reps
half squat	0	5	0	5	0	5	0	5	5	3	5	3
reverse lunge	0	5	0	5	0	5	0	5	5	3	5	3
bicep curl-up	2	5	2	5	2	10	2	10	5	5	5	5
tricep kickback	2	5	2	5	2	10	2	10	5	5	5	5
wall push-up		5		5		6	6			7		7
abdominal curl		5		5		6	6			6		6
balance	15s		15s		15s		15s		20s		20s	

NOTES

EVALUATE YOUR FOOD PREFERENCES

Instructions:
- Fill in the points in the right column, for each food.
- Total the points for each section (Vegetables, Fruits, Grains and Fats).

What the score means:
- Approximate dividing lines:
    - o Vegetables and Fruits: 100 points each
    - o Grains: 30 points
    - o Fats: 20 points
- A score above these numbers simply means you're open to a wide variety of foods and should have an easy time with the Battle of Quality.
- A score below these numbers doesn't mean that *Resetting Normal* won't work for you, just that you may have more limited choices for your selection of quality foods. The chart below is available in the workbook on the website ***resettingnormal.com***, if you want to print it.

Description	Points
Love it!	5
Like it	4
It's ok—wouldn't refuse it but not wild about it	3
Don't know—willing to try it	2
Have never liked it, but willing to try a different preparation	1
Hate it—you couldn't pay me to eat it	0
VEGETABLES	**Points**
Asparagus	
Avocado	
Beans, green (string)	
Beans, dried (black, kidney, red, pinto, white, etc.)	
Beets	
Broccoli	
Brussels sprouts	
Cabbage (red, green, Savoy, napa, etc.)	
Carrots	
Cauliflower	
Celery	
Corn	

Cucumber	
Edamame (fresh soybeans)	
Eggplant	
Garlic	
Ginger	
Greens (kale, endive, beet, collard, mustard, chard, etc.)	
Kohlrabi	
Lettuce (iceberg)	
Lettuce (looseleaf, bibb, Romaine, etc.)	
Mushrooms	
Okra	
Onions	
Parsnips	
Peas	
Peppers (hot)	
Peppers (sweet)	
Potatoes (regular)	
Potatoes (sweet, yams)	
Radishes	
Spinach	
Tomatoes	
Turnips or rutabagas	
Squash (winter—orange)	
Squash (summer—zucchini, yellow, etc.)	
TOTAL	
FRUITS	**Points**
Apple	
Apricot	
Asian Pear	
Banana/Plantain	
Blackberries	
Blueberries	
Cactus Pear	
Cantaloupe	
Cherries	
Coconut	
Cranberries	
Currants	
Dates	

Figs	
Grapes	
Grapefruit/Pomelo	
Guava	
Honeydew Melon	
Kiwifruit	
Lemons	
Limes	
Mangoes	
Nectarines	
Oranges	
Papaya	
Passion Fruit	
Peaches	
Pears	
Pineapple	
Plums	
Pomegranate	
Raspberries	
Strawberries	
Tangerines	
Watermelon	
TOTAL	
GRAINS	**Points**
Bulgur	
Millet	
Multigrain cereal (cooked)	
Quinoa	
Rice, brown	
Rice, wild	
Unsweetened regular oatmeal	
Unsweetened whole wheat cereals (cold), such as Shredded Wheat	
Whole wheat bread (loaf, pita, wraps, etc.)	
Whole wheat cereal (cooked)	
Whole wheat pasta	
TOTAL	

FATS	Points
Butter	
Flax oil	
Lard	
Olive oil	
Safflower oil	
Sesame oil	
Vegetable oil (canola, corn)	
TOTAL	

SEE WHAT YOU ACTUALLY EAT

For the Battle of Quality, Action #7

If last week was typical of the meals you usually eat, write down approximately what you ate. If it wasn't (maybe you were on vacation or there was something special going on) then choose the last week that was typical. You don't have to be too specific. Below is an example.

Meal/snack	Day of the week	Day of week	...
	Monday	Tuesday	...
Breakfast	OJ; scrambled eggs; toast with butter; coffee	Protein bar; coffee	
Snack	...	Strawberry yogurt	
Lunch	2 slices pizza with pepperoni; Diet soda	2 fast-food chicken tacos; French fries; Diet soda	
Snack	Raw carrots	...	
Dinner	2 pieces ready-made roast chicken; small salad with low-fat Caesar Dressing; Frozen French fries; 2 cookies; Diet soda	2 slices meatloaf; mac & cheese; string beans; ice cream; water	
Snack	Small bowl tortilla chips with salsa	Diet soda	

This exercise will give you a good idea of how much processed food vs. real food you already eat.

EVALUATE YOUR CURRENT FOOD SUPPLY

For the Battle of Quality, Action #8

Using the sample chart below, make a list of twelve products in your pantry/fridge/freezer that you use the most. For each product on your list, read the ingredients on the label. Based on the number of additives and/or preservatives, check the appropriate column on the chart. Then in the last column enter the amount of sugar. You don't have to record the number of additives/preservatives, but I did in the sample just to enhance the information for you.

- Whole: two or fewer
- In-between: three to five
- Highly processed: more than five
- Sugar: number of grams

If you're unsure about which ingredients qualify, see the *Appendix C: Additives and Preservatives*.

The additive monosodium glutamate (MSG) deserves special attention because its safety is controversial. The FDA considers it safe, but many nutritionists do not. It occurs naturally in some foods, such as tomatoes, cheeses, and many proteins. But most food products that contain it come from chemically produced sources. Seaweed is particularly high in glutamate content, and that was the original source from which Kikunae Ikeda extracted glutamate and patented it for commercial production in 1908. Some people are sensitive to it and others don't seem to be—at least not in the short term.

My take on this additive is to be cautious and remember that the package matters. While seaweed may have lots of naturally occurring MSG, it may also have all the associated enzymes and other digestive helpers for your body to metabolize it properly. Extracting MSG and adding it in unknown quantities to practically every food product out there doesn't take that into account, and may well lead to an overload that could cause health problems over time. As MSG has many different names, I've included a list of the more common ones in the *Appendix C*.

A note on added sugars: this is hard to calculate because food labeling doesn't separate naturally occurring sugar from added sugar. For instance, the sugar in flavored yogurt includes the natural sugar in milk (lactose), plus the natural sugar in fruit, plus additional sugars to sweeten the yogurt overall. Until the labeling changes, the only way to evaluate a product is to consider the total. Since that total is given in grams—which isn't very meaningful—you can do a simple conversion to get a better picture of the amount of sugar in the product.

- 4 grams = 1 teaspoon
- 12 grams = 3 teaspoons = 1 Tablespoon
- 48 grams = 4 Tablespoons = ¼ cup

Example: To get the number of teaspoons of sugar in a product that contains 8 grams of sugar, divide the 8 grams by 4 and you get 2 teaspoons.

Product	Whole: 2 or fewer	In-between: 3-5	Highly processed: more than 5	Sugar
Canned tomatoes	✓ (2)			0 grams
Cup O'Noodles Chicken Flavor			✓ (19)	2 grams per package
Doritos: Nacho Flavor			✓ (11)	0 grams
Healthy Choice Grilled Chicken Pesto with Vegetables			✓ (13)	2 grams per package
Heinz Chili Sauce		✓ (4)		3 grams per Tablespoon
Keebler Coconut Dreams			✓ (13)	10 grams (2½ teaspoons) per 2 cookies
Miracle Whip Light			✓ (9)	Less than 2 grams, but has artificial sweeteners
Nestle Vanilla Fudge Drumstick			✓ (18)	24 grams (2 Tablespoons) per drumstick
Orowheat 100% Whole Wheat Bread		✓ (7)		3 grams (less than 1 teaspoon) per slice
Quaker Instant Oats: Apple flavored			✓ (6)	12 grams (1 Tablespoon) per package
String beans: frozen	✓ (0)			0 grams
Triscuits	✓ (0)			0 grams
Wheaties	✓ (1)			4 grams per ¾ cup (1 teaspoon)
Yoplait Original Yogurt Raspberry		✓ (4)		18 grams (1½ Tablespoons) per package

This Action should give you a good idea how much processed food you commonly use and where to start making changes—look to the third and fourth columns for the worst offenders.

NOTES

APPENDIX C: ADDITIVES AND PRESERVATIVES
Vitamins

A number of processed foods have added vitamins and minerals—many required by government regulation. Frequently they are listed in parentheses by their chemical names. Although they do indicate that a product has been refined (its original nutrients removed by processing), you don't need to avoid them. If you see any of the following names in a product's ingredient list, *don't count* them as additives.

Chemical Names	Vitamin	Chemical Names	Vitamin	Chemical Names	Vitamin
Beta-carotene, Retinol	A	Pyradoxine	B6	Vitamin D2 (ergocalciferol)	D
Thiamine, Thiamin	B1	Biotin	B7	Vitamin D3 (cholecalciferol)	D
Riboflavin	B2	Folic acid, Folate	B9	Tocopherol	E
Niacin, Nicotinic acid, Niacinamide	B3	Cyanocobalamin, Methylcobalamin	B12		
Pantothenic acid	B5	Ascorbic acid	C		

Added sugars

COMMON NAMES

The USDA website *choosemyplate.gov/what-are-added-sugars* lists the following as added sugars:
- anhydrous dextrose
- brown sugar
- confectioner's powdered sugar
- corn syrup
- corn-syrup solids
- dextrose
- fructose
- high-fructose corn syrup (HFCS)
- honey
- invert sugar
- lactose
- malt syrup
- maltose
- maple syrup
- molasses
- nectars (e.g., peach nectar, pear nectar)
- pancake syrup
- raw sugar
- sucrose
- sugar

The website also lists the following as unofficial (not recognized by the FDA) names for added sugars:
- cane juice or evaporated cane juice
- evaporated corn sweetener
- crystal dextrose
- glucose
- liquid fructose
- sugar-cane juice

Common artificial sweeteners

- Acesulfame potassium
- Aspartame (Equal, Nutrasweet)
- Erythritol
- Maltitol
- Mannitol
- Neotame
- Saccharin (Sugar Twin, Sweet'N Low)
- Sucralose (Splenda)
- Sorbitol
- Xylitol

Common food additives and preservatives

- Butylated hydroxyanisole (BHA)
- Butylated hydroxytoluene (BHT)
- Calcium carbonate
- Carrageenan
- Erythorbic acid
- Glycerin
- Guar gum
- Lactic acid
- Lecithin
- Methylcellulose
- Mono- and Diglycerides
- Monosodium Glutamate (MSG)
- Pectin
- Phosphoric acid
- Potassium bisulfite
- Potassium metabisulfite
- Potassium nitrate
- Sodium aluminosilicate
- Sodium benzoate
- Sodium bisulfite
- Sodium metabisulfite
- Sodium nitrite
- Sodium sulfite
- Sulfur dioxide

Alternate names for Monosodium Glutamate (MSG)

MSG occurs in some foods naturally, such as tomatoes, cheeses, seaweed, and others. But the MSG in most food products is produced chemically and goes by many names. Below are some of the most common ones:

- Textured protein
- Autolyzed yeast (extract)
- Autolyzed plant protein
- Calcium caseinate
- Hydrolyzed plant protein (HPP)
- Natural flavors (may or may not contain MSG)
- Sodium caseinate
- Glutamate
- Glutamic Acid
- Hydrolyzed protein
- Hydrolyzed vegetable protein (HVP)
- Soy protein extract
- Soy protein isolate
- Yeast extract
- Yeast food

APPENDIX D: ADDITIONAL READING

The following groups of books provide additional background information on the state of our Western food lifestyle and potential modifications that can make it better. Some are more technical than others, but I list them here in case you want to explore these ideas.

FOOD AND NUTRITION

Davis, Adelle. *Let's Eat Right to Keep Fit.* New York: Harcourt, Brace Jovanovich, Inc, 1954.

Dufty, William. *Sugar Blues.* New York: Warner Books, 1975.

Gittleman, Ann Louise and J. Lynne Dodson. *Super Nutrition for Women: A Food-Wise Guide for Health, Beauty, Energy, and Immunity.* New York: Bantam Books, 1991.

Gittleman, Ann Louise with J. Maxwell Desgrey. *Beyond Pritikin.* New York: Bantam Books, 1988.

Planck, Nina. *Real Food: What to eat and why.* New York: Bloomsbury USA, 2006.

Pollan, Michael. *In Defense of Food: An Eater's Manifesto.* New York: The Penguin Press, 2008.

—. The Omnivore's Dilemma: *A Natural History of Four Meals.* New York: Penguin Books, 2006.

Robinson, Jo. *Eating on the Wild Side: The Missing Link to Optimum Health.* New York: Little, Brown and Company, 2013.

WEIGHT

Bacon, Linda. *Health at Every Size: The surprising truth about your weight.* Dallas: BenBella Books, Inc., 2008.[10]

Clower, Dr. Will. *The Fat Fallacy: The French Diet Secrets to Permanent Weight Loss.* New York: Three Rivers Press, 2003.

Kolata, Gina. *Rethinking Thin: The New Science of Weight Loss—and the Myths and Realities of Dieting* New York: Picador, 2007.

Taubes, Gary. *Good Calories. Bad Calories: Challenging the Conventional Wisdom on Diet, Weight Control, and Disease.* New York: Alfred A. Knopf, 2007.

EXERCISE

Pagano, Joan. *Strength Training Exercises for Women.* New York: DK, 2013.

Yeager, Selene, and Editors of Women's Health. *The Women's Health Big Book of 15-Minute Workouts.* New York: Rodale, 2011.

Yeager, Selene, and Editors of Men's Health. *The Men's Health Big Book of 15-Minute Workouts.* New York: Rodale, 2011.

Perkins, Holly. *Women's Health Lift to Get Lean: A Beginner's Guide to Fitness & Strength Training in 3 Simple Steps.* New York, Rodale Inc, 2015.

Lauren, Mark, and Joshua Clark. *You Are Your Own Gym: The Bible of Bodyweight Exercises.* New York: Ballentine Books, 2011.

Fox, Abby. *Weight Training (Idiot's Guides).* New York: Penguin Group (USA) Inc, 2013.Campbell, Adam. *The Women's Health Little Book of Exercises: Four Weeks to a Leaner, Sexier, Healthier You!.* New York: Rodale Inc, 2014.

Schlosberg, Suzanne, and Liz Neporent. *Fitness for Dummies.* Indiana, Wiley Publishing, Inc., 2010.

Swanson, Larry. *Scared Sitless: The Office Fitness Book.* Seattle, Elless Media, LLC, 2014.

THE FOOD INDUSTRY

Brownell, Kelly D. and Katherine Battle Horgen. *Food Fight: The Inside Story of the Food Industry, America's Obesity Crisis & What We Can Do About It.* McGraw-Hill, 2004.

Estabrook, Barry. *Tomatoland.* Kansas City: Andrews McMeel Publishing, LLC, 2011.

Kessler, David A. *The End of Overeating: Taking Control of the Insatiable American Appetite.* New York: Rodale, 2009.

Ogle, Maureen. *In Meat We Trust.* New York: Houghton Mifflin Harcourt Publishing Company, 2013.

Oliver, J. Eric. *Fat Politics: The Real Story Behind America's Obesity Epidemic.* Ebook. Oxford University Press, 2005.

Nestle, Marion. *Food Politics: How the Food Industry Influences Nutrition and Health.* Berkeley: University of California Press, Ltd., 2007.

Patel, Raj. *Stuffed and Starved: The Hidden Battle for the World Food System.* Ebook. Melville House, 2012.

Roberts, Paul. *The End of Food.* New York: Houghton Mifflin, 2008.

Simon, Michele. *Appetite for Profit: How the Food Industry Undermines our Health and How to Fight Back.* Ebook. Nation Books, 2009.

Weber, Karl. *Food, Inc.: A Participant Guide: How Industrial Food is Making us Sicker, Fatter, and Poorer—And What You Can Do About It.* Ebook. PublicAffairs, 2009.

BACKGROUND

Buettner, Dan. *The Blue Zones: Lessons for Living Longer From the People Who've Lived the Longest.* Washington, D.C.: National Geographic Society, 2008.

Daniel, Kaayla T. *The Whole Soy Story: The Dark Side of America's Favorite Health Food.* NewTrends Publishing, Inc., 2005.

Doidge, Norman. *The Brain that Changes Itself.* New York: Penguin Group, 2007.
Fitzgerald, Randall. *The Hundred-Year Lie: How Food and Medicine are Destroying Your Health.* Dutton Adult, 2006

Freedman, David H. *Wrong: Why Experts* Keep Failing Us and How to Know When Not to Trust Them.* New York: Little, Brown and Company, 2010.

Rothstein, William G. *Public Health and the Risk Factor: A History of an Uneven Medical Revolution.* Rochester: University of Rochester Press, 2003.

Wrangham, Richard. *Catching Fire: How Cooking Made Us Human.* New York: Basic Books, 2009.

CHEMISTRY

Buist, Robert. *Food Chemical Sensitivity.* Garden City Park: Avery Publishing Group, Inc., 1986.

Enig, Mary G. *Know Your Fats: The Complete Guide for Understanding the Nutrition of Fats, Oils, and Cholesterol.* Bethesda: Bethesda Press, 2015.

Erasmus, Udo. *Fats that Heal—Fats that Kill.* Burnaby: Alive Books, 1996. Reference

Gilman, Sander L. *Diets and Dieting: A Cultural Encyclopedia.* Ebook. Routledge, 2008.

Winter, Ruth. *A Consumer's Dictionary of Food Additives.* 7. New York: Harmony, 2009.

ENDNOTES

1. Freedman, David H. Wrong: *Why Experts* Keep Failing Us* and *How to Know When Not to Trust Them.* (New York: Little, Brown and Company, 2010), Introduction.

2. Cameron, Robert. *The Drinking Man's Diet.* Cameron + Company, 1964.

3. Powter, Susan. *Stop the Insanity!.* New York: Simon & Schuster Inc., 1993.

4. Atkins, Robert C. Dr. Atkins' *Diet Revolution.* Bantam, 1981.

5. Sears, Barry. *Enter the Zone.* Regan Book, 1995.

6. Simpson, Jerry H., Jr. "Joke." *Reader's Digest. Laughter: The Best Medicine.* Pleasantville: Reader's Digest Trade Publishing, 2008. 212.

7. Swinburn, Boyd. "Boyd Swinburn: combating obesity at the community level." The Lancet 378.9793 (2011): 761.

8. Kolata, Gina. After-'The Biggest Loser,' *Their Bodies Fought to Gain Weight. Investigative Journalism.* New York: The New York Times, 2016. Website. ***www.newyorktimes.com/2016/05/02/health/biggest-loser-weight-loss.html?emc=etal&_r=0.***

9. Kelly, Walt. Pogo: *We Have Met the Enemy and He is Us.* 2nd Printing edition (November 1987). New York: Simon & Schuster, 1987.

10. Moore, Thomas J. Lifespan: *Who Lives Longer and Why.* New York: Simon & Schuster, 1993.

11. Bacon, Linda. *Health at Every Size: The surprising truth about your weight.* Dallas: BenBella Books, Inc., 2008.

12. Sears, Barry. *Enter the Zone.* (Regan Book, 1995), pp. 14 – 18.

13. Erasmus, Udo. *Fats that Heal – Fats that Kill.* (Burnaby: Alive Books, 1996), chap. 6.

14. Nestle, Marion. Food Politics: *How the Food Industry Influences Nutrition and Health.* (University of California Press, Ltd., 2007), pp. 239 – 246.

15. Powter, Susan. *Stop the Insanity!* (New York: Simon & Schuster Inc., 1993), pp. 161.

16. Ogle, Maureen. *In Meat We Trust.* (New York: Houghton Mifflin Harcourt Publishing Company, 2013), pp. 223 – 261.

17. Doidge, Norman. *The Brain that Changes Itself.* (New York: Penguin Group, 2007), pp. 168 – 174.

18. Kessler, David. *The End of Overeating: Taking Control of the Insatiable American Appetite* New York: Rodale, 2009.

19. Estabrook, Barry. T*omatoland.* Kansas City: Andrews McMeel Publishing, LLC, 2011.

INDEX

80/20 principle, **38**
  for convenience, **134**
  for processed foods, **116**
  in social situations, **66**

A

activity
  aerobic, **86 – 93**
  barriers to, **73, 77 - 79**
  benefits of, **72**
  blockage, **73 - 75**
  burnout, **74 – 75**
  charts, **230, 234**
  discouragements, **79 – 81**
  everyday, **73, 81 - 86**
  vs. exercise, **73**
  goals, **74 - 75**
  and Western Lifestyle, **29**
  in Resetting Normal, **37**
  importance of, **70 - 72**
  on holidays, vacations, travel, **90**
  for kids, **208**
  mini-activities, **81 - 86**
  physical assessment for, **74**
  Pilates, **99 - 100**
  safest, **75**
  strength, **93 - 100**
  types of, **73**
  and weight loss, **47, 70, 79**
additives, **243-244**
  acceptable, **117, 243**
  cumulative effect of, **121**
  FDA approval of, **65, 113, 244**
  and gut bacteria, **154 - 155**
  in evaluating your food supply, **240**
  in low-fat products, **53, 110, 126**
  in processed foods, **113, 119**
  reference book, **113**
  relationship to "fresh", **114 - 115**
  in seasonings, **211**
Adele Davis, **31**
Adobo seasoning, Mexican, recipe, **213**
advertising, **65**
  claims, **65**
aerobic
  activities, **86 - 93**
  American Heart Association recommendations, **89**
  barriers to, **73, 77 - 79**
  benefits of, **72**
  and breathing, **86, 87**
  and mental processes, **86**
  definition of, **86**
  discouragements, **79 - 80**
  how to increase, **92**
  and weight loss, **79**
affirmations, **75**
agriculture, **27, 109**
alcohol
  Drinking Man's Diet, **15**
  effect on appetite, **180, 194**
appestat
  broken, **158-159**
  definition of, **24**
  internal, **0, 31, 38, 40, 43, 55, 125, 161, 195**
appetite

and alcohol, **180, 194**
and fat, **146 - 148**
and food cravings, **100, 102, 127, 143, 154**
and gut bacteria, **154**
and gremlin, **48 - 50**
and the "package", **108 - 109**
regulation of, **24, 43, 106, 118, 124, 148**
satisfaction, **21, 106, 109 - 111, 164 - 165, 169 - 170**
signals, **27**
and sleep, **100 - 103**
and whole foods, **106 - 107**
Apricots, Rehydrated, **226**
artificial sweeteners, **244**
  in cereals, **113**
  for kids, **207**
  in low-fat products, **53**
  in smoothies, **123**
Atkins Diet, **15, 17, 165**

B

balance
  in appetite regulation, **109-110**
  and cravings, **165**
  of food types, **165 – 166, 193 - 194**
  hormone theory, **175**
  in meal planning, **193 - 194**
  in physical fitness, **84, 87, 93**
  for weight loss, **193**
  in the Zone Diet, **18, 165**
barriers
  identifying, **77 - 79**
  to movement, **73**
  overcoming, **77 - 79**
  to sleep, **101**
baseline
  for Final Frontier, **190**
  for physical activity, **76, 97**
Bean and Bacon Soup, recipe, **225**
beef, **53, 115**
  ground, Unboxed Dinner, recipe, **219**
binge
  defusing, **53**
  preventing, **54**
blindfold test, **168 - 169**
Blueberry Freeze, recipe, **226**
BMI, **74**
body mass index, **74**
boxed mixes, ways to replace, **149 - 150**
breakfast
  when to eat, **54, 56**
  what to eat, **143, 147, 164**
  for children, **207**
  Breakfast Ideas, **215 - 217**
  Breakfast Muffins, recipe, **215**
  business travel, **185, 187**
buzzwords, **129 - 131**

C

cake recipes
  Cocoa, **227**
  Vanilla, **228**
  Spice, **229**
  Lemon, **229**

  Orange, **229**
calories
  counting, **45**
  burning, **47 - 49**
  definition, **47**
  vs. nutritional values, **45, 66**
  in/out theory, **47 – 49, 79**
carbohydrates/carb/carbs
  Atkins Diet, **17**
  balancing, **193 - 195**
  cravings, **102, 154, 165**
  Drinking Man's Diet, **15**
  effect on appetite, **143, 147**
  excess, **63**
  refined and gut bacteria, **154**
  and low-fat diet, **17**
  measurement on exercise machines, **89**
  vs. nutritional value, **45**
cat metaphor, **169 - 171**
cereal alternatives, **215**
chemistry, **108**
Chicken in a Flash, recipe, **222**
clear-the-deck mentality, **65, 129 - 136, 207**
Cocoa Cake, recipe, **227**
commercial-proof, **65, 129 - 136, 207**
comparison
  calorie, **147**
  portion envy, **174 - 175**
  real cupcakes vs. processed, **118 – 119**
  Resetting Normal vs. diets, **40**
convenience foods, **29, 34, 83, 121, 134, 144 - 145**
conventional wisdom, **62 - 64**
cycle, denial-indulgence, **33, 37, 47, 50, 52, 69**

D

Davis, Adelle, **31**
denial, and indulgence cycle, **33, 37, 47, 50, 52, 69**
deprivation, perception of, **167 - 175**
deprogramming, **20 – 22**
diet, dieting, diets
  1960s, **14**
  Atkins, **17**
  author's personal history of, **13 – 19**
  balance, **165 - 167**
  body-type, **17**
  comparison with Resetting Normal, **40**
  cottage cheese and peaches, **14**
  cycle of, **14**
  description of, **7**
  Drinking Man's, **15**
  failure of, **7, 46 - 49**
  food patterns, **122 – 123**
  and gut bacteria, **154**
  low-carbohydrate, **15, 17**
  low-fat, **17**
  maintenance, **7, 36, 42**
  mentality, **20, 39, 58, 64**
  obsessed culture, **30**
  paradox, **50**

249

paradigm, 27, 50
societal cycles of, 10
Western, 29, 34
yo-yo, 7
The Zone, 18
diet-proof, 46 – 61
kids, 207
diet industry, 33
diet math, 47 - 49
diet soda, 126, 132
Dinners, Unboxed, recipes, 219 – 223
discouragements, 79 - 81
disorders, eating, 30

E

endurance, aerobic, 73, 86
equipment
cooking, 200
strength training, 97 - 99
everyday activity, 81 - 86
exercise
and weight loss, 37, 40, 48, 70
in Resetting Normal, 40
importance of, 70
benefits of, 72
barriers to, 73, 77 – 79
mini, 81 – 86
aerobic, suggestions, 91
Pilates, 99 - 100
expert, definition of, 10
expert-proof, 61 – 65
extrapolation, fallacy of, 152 - 155

F

family, influence of, 13, 32, 68, 159, 205
farm-raised, 122, 198
farmers' market, 116, 198
fat
hydrogenated, 31
calories in, 47
1980s advice, 61
and satisfaction, 110
saturated, 63, 124, 126
to replace sugar, 146 - 147
FDA, 65, 113, 121, 239
feedback, 55, 95
loop, 162 - 163, 171, 177
Fish Dinner, 220
fitness, evaluation, 74
food drought, 57 - 58
Food and Drug Administration, 113
See also FDA
food industry, 29 – 30, 31, 65, 110, 111, 115, 11 – 118, 120, 121, 125, 126, 129
deals, 183 - 185
food preferences, 137, 142, 152, 235 - 238
food supply, evaluation, 131, 136, 138, 238 - 241
freshness, in quality food, 114 – 115

G

Goldilocks, 160 - 167
gremlin, 48 – 50
Ground Meat Dinner, recipe, 219
gut bacteria, 154
gym, equipment, 99

H

health-nut, aura, 67
help, 144 - 151
holidays, vacation, travel, 185 - 188
homeostasis, 47, 185, 186, 191
hormones
body, 70, 72, 175
in food, 115, 118

I

indulgence, denial and, 33, 37, 47, 50, 52, 69
Italian seasoning, recipe, 213

J

junk food, 106, 120, 122, 144, 154, 204, 205

K

kids, 85, 131, 159, 203 - 209

L

label, reading, 66, 124
chart, 130
Lemon Cake, recipe, 229
low-calorie, 126, 183
trap, 132
low-carb/low-carbohydrate, diet, 15, 17
low-fat
craziness, 125 – 126
diet, 17
foods, 31, 110
trap, 132

M

mac and cheese, 60, 67, 147, 149, 161
Mac & Cheese, recipe, 221
Marketing Machine, 129 – 136, 184
Battle of Activity, 104
Battle of the Mind, 68
Battle of Quality, 155
Battle of Quantity, 188
Final Frontier, 195
media, influence of, 11, 32 -33
menopause, 18, 176
metabolic, 21, 40, 48, 61, 130, 153, 154, 161, 165, 170
conversation, imaginary, 186
gremlin, 48 – 50
plumbing, 109
metabolism, 27, 28, 47 – 49, 55, 63, 64, 72, 106, 108, 109, 123, 150, 153 – 155, 175, 185
and age, 174
metaphor, 185 - 187
metaphor
cat, 169 – 170
Goldilocks, 160
for homeostasis, 185 - 187
for Resetting Normal, 28, 35
Mexican Adobo seasoning, recipe, 213
mind and body, partnership, 50, 143
Minestrone, Easy, recipe, 223
mini-activities, 81 – 86
monosodium glutamate, 113, 120, See also MSG
MSG, 113, 120, 239, 244

N

NASCAR eater, 179

natural
food processing, 117
all-natural, trap, 132, 134
in labeling, 132
non-fat, 53, 110, 126, 132
trap, 132
nutrition, nutritional, 45, 66, 106, 112, 114,117, 122, 123, 125, 128,150, 159, 179, 183, 185, 199, 201, 205, 210
nutritionist, 31, 47, 48, 65, 239

O

obesity, 7, 27, 28, 31, 46, 132, 203, 204, 205, 209
obesogenic, 28, 204
omnivore, 42, 122
Orange Cake, recipe, 229
organic, 66, 116, 122, 130, 197
overeat, overeating, 10, 110, 147, 157,158, 162, 169, 172, 177, 178, 185, 195

P

the package matters, 108 - 109
perception, 24, 77, 135, 161, 167, 170, 180
kids', 203, 206, 209
recalibrate, 167 – 178
permission to eat, 20, 51 - 53
pharmaceutical industry, 33
Pilaf from scratch, 214
Pilates, 95, 99
Pima Indians, 28
pleasure principle, 136
Pogo, 33 - 35
portion envy, 174 - 175
Power of One, 171 - 173
preservatives, 112, 113, 114, 118, 120, 121, 243 - 245
and gut bacteria, 154
on labels, 113, 131
in salad dressings, 217
in spice mixes, 212
processed food, 229, 30, 34, 38, 42, 51, 53, 58, 67, 69, 101, 110, 112, 116,120, 121, 129, 133, 141, 150, 158, 159, 168, 178, 181, 197
how to identify, 116 – 119
in limited budget, 181
role in snacktivity, 168, 169
protein, 110 – 111, 115, 123, 127, 130, 143, 151, 167, 186, 192, 194, 198
in balanced meals, 143, 193
soy, 123, 127, 130

Q

quality
Battle of, defined, 37, 106
in body chemistry, 108
foods, 30, 37, 106, 111 – 116, 198 - 200, 235 - 238
vs. quantity, 22, 24, 38, 61, 106, 111, 126, 154, 163, 168, 176, 183
Resetting Normal vs. diets, 40
of your rest, 102
quantity, 20, 21, 22, 36, 118
Battle of, defined, 38, 156
−conscious, 180-181

250

feedback, **163**
food types, **193**
forGoldilocks, **162**
for kids, **206, 209**
in low-fat diet, **17**
perception of, **167 - 168**
vs. quality, **38, 106, 111, 152, 163, 174, 183**
Resetting Normal vs. diets, **40**
and satisfaction, **111, 169, 176, 183**
trap, **133**

R

real food, **25, 38, 56, 109, 115 – 116, 118, 123, 125, 138, 198**
definition of, **115**
refined
carbohydrates, **31, 53, 101, 102, 110, 141, 145 - 146**
craving, **101 - 102**
grains, **145 - 146**
and gut bacteria, **154**
for kids, **206**
RESET, **38, 138 - 139, 140, 143, 194**
resistance bands, **94, 95, 96, 97, 98**
restaurant, **15, 18, 134, 144, 148, 149, 151, 171, 184 – 185, 197, 204, 205**
restrictive eating, **16, 17, 51, 52**
reward, food as, **52, 54, 60, 204, 206**
rules, **47, 52, 55, 56, 57, 62**
for everyday activities, **81**
for the Final Frontier, **190, 192**
for RESET, **136**

S

salad dressing
Oil and Lemon, recipe, **218**
Oil and Vinegar, recipe, **217**
problem, **148**
Ranch-style, recipe, **218**
satisfaction, **21, 39, 40, 106, 109 - 111, 125, 127, 164, 165, 168, 169 - 170, 175, 179, 183, 184, 189**
factor, **109 - 111**
potential, **106**
and quantity, **169 - 170**
in *Resetting Normal*, **40**
saturated fat, **52, 63, 124, 126 - 127, 148, 149**
scale, **44 – 45, 188, 190, 210**
seasoning, **120, 150, 211 – 213**
Basic list, **212 - 213**
Italian, recipe, **213**
Mexican Adobo, recipe, **213**
Morton & Bassett, **212**
Penzeys, **212**
Simply Organic, **212**
silver bullet, **34, 123**
sleep, **100 - 104**
and food cravings, **101, 102, 147**
slow cooker, **145, 200**
Minestrone, **223**
Bean and Bacon Soup, **225**
smoothies, **123 - 124**
snacktivity, **183**
social context, **178 - 182**
social-proof, **66 - 68**
soup
Minestrone, Easy, recipe, **223**
Bean and Bacon, recipe, **225**
Southwest Breakfast Muffins, recipe, **215**
soy, **64, 112, 120, 127, 133, 151, 217**
Spice Cake, recipe, **229**
spices, **116, 149, 198, 200**
See also seasonings
strength, **71, 73, 76**
training, **76, 93 - 100**
sugar, **14, 31, 54, 58, 63, 66, 101, 111, 112, 115, 116, 117, 120, 131,145, 142, 154, 159**
and kids, **206 - 207**
ways to replace, **146 – 148**
supermarket shortcuts, **144 - 145**
sweetener, **53, 110, 112, 123, 125, 131, 136, 148, 207, 244**
artificial, **53, 123, 131, 207, 244**
stevia, **116**

T

Tacos, recipe, **220**
theory, **18, 47, 62**
on aging, and exercise, **72 - 73, 86**
on aging, and weight, **175**
on cravings, **154**
on gut bacteria,**154**
on overeating, **157 – 158**
thin = healthy, **27, 46, 63**
trans-fat, **31, 126, 148**
trap, bear, **131 - 136**
travel, holidays, vacation, **185 - 188**
treadmill math, **89**

U

United States Department of Agriculture, **194**
See also USDA
unprocessed foods, **117**
USDA, **194**

V

vacation, travel, holidays, **185 - 188**
Vanilla Cake, recipe, **228**
vegan, **42, 120, 122, 127, 130 40, 112, 113, 119**
trap, **133**
vegetarian, **42, 63, 120, 122, 127, 167, 194**
trap, **133**

W

Western lifestyle, **8, 29, 34, 46, 67, 181 - 182, 203**
managing, **181 - 182**
theory, **154**
workbook, **16, 45, 76, 77, 79, 92, 98, 100, 138, 142, 162, 163**
walking, **13, 20, 23, 72, 76, 78, 80, 83, 85, 86, 87, 88, 90, 91, 92, 93, 188, 208**
we are what we eat, **34, 107, 153**
weights, **73, 93, 94, 95, 96, 98, 98, 100**
whole-foods advantage, **106 - 111**
weight-loss, **45, 50**
trap, **135**
weight, soft, **186 - 187**
weight, hard, **186 - 187**
whole grain, **31, 108, 115, 130, 145, 146, 198, 199, 201, 214, 215**
whole-grain, **66, 113, 141, 145, 167, 182, 200, 201, 206, 214**
whole grains, easy, recipes, **214**
Whole-Food Alternatives, **211**

X

Y

yo-yo, dieter, **7, 8, 44, 58, 69**
yo-yo, exercising, **74, 77**
yo-yobesity, **7, 9, 12, 15, 16, 19, 21, 25, 37, 46, 47, 50, 59, 69, 156, 207, 209, 210**
you are what you eat, **107 - 109**
Yogurt, recipe, **216**

Z

The Zone, diet, **18, 165**
zoo, metaphor, **28**

ABOUT THE AUTHOR

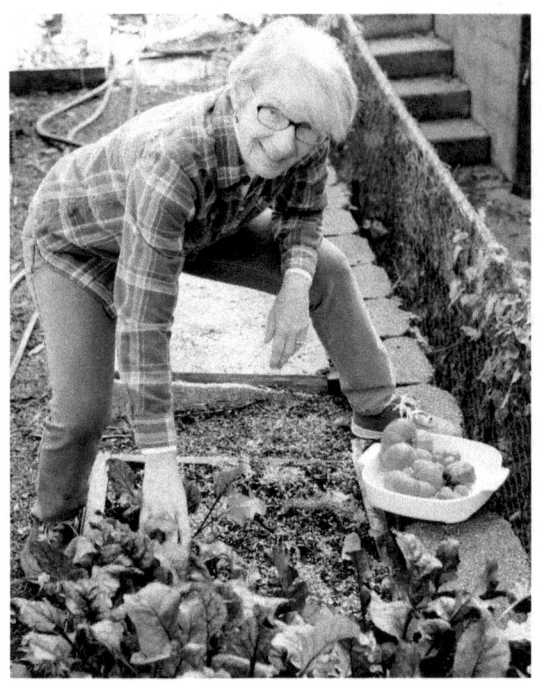

Research shows that over time, yo-yo dieters - the people who try every diet program out there but never find one that sticks – typically gain more weight than they lose.

Tessa Wizon was one of those people until she found a way to break the pattern. Abandoning standard weight loss advice, Tessa devised a fresh approach that helped her lose the weight she wanted and keep it off for over 12 years.

Resetting Normal offers Tessa's unique method and provides yo-yo dieters with an achievable action plan to end their yo-yobesity – that gradual weight gain that results when the dieting cycle's up-the-scale exceeds down-the-scale. Tessa shows how you can attack and defeat the real underlying causes of yo-yobesity by winning four battles - the Battle of the Mind, the Battle of Activity, the Battle of Quality, and the Battle of Quantity.

This is not a diet book! Tessa's approach will remove all dietary stress from your life. You won't need to count calories, fat grams, carbs or anything else. You won't gain weight from holidays or vacations. No diets, no scale, no BMI calculations. For yo-yo dieters who want to escape the endless cycle of weight gain and disappointment, this is a completely different way to normalize your weight without dieting and effortlessly keep it stable for the rest of your life.

www.ingramcontent.com/pod-product-compliance
Lightning Source LLC
Chambersburg PA
CBHW070917030426
42336CB00014BA/2455